The FORGIVENESS Diet

A Healing Guide for African-American Women
and the People Who Love Them

The FORGIVENESS Diet

*How to Lose the Weight
and Keep it Off*

by Dr. Jendayo Grady

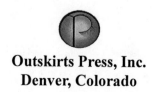

Outskirts Press, Inc.
Denver, Colorado

The Forgiveness Diet
How to Lose the Weight and Keep it Off
A Healing Guide for African-American Women and the People Who Love Them
All Rights Reserved.
Copyright © 2011 Dr. Jendayo Grady
v2.0 r1.0

Outskirts Press, Inc.
http://www.outskirtspress.com

ISBN: 978-1-4327-7599-5

Outskirts Press and the "OP" logo are trademarks belonging to Outskirts Press, Inc.

PRINTED IN THE UNITED STATES OF AMERICA

This book is dedicated to the scores of resilient women who have labored incessantly, yet are still broken. It is now time for you to be restored and healed!

God Bless You!

ACKNOWLEDGMENTS

I want to acknowledge the following persons:

- Thank You Heavenly Father for adopting me into Your loving care. Thank You for teaching me how to acknowledge You in all my ways.
- Thank You Lord Jesus for shedding Your blood for me, whereby I could be forgiven.
- Thank You Holy Spirit for giving me new life and leading me to my destiny.
- I want to acknowledge my wonderful, wise, and beautiful wife, Kellie. Your undying love, wisdom, support, and sacrifice have blessed me in ways that words cannot express. You truly are my better half! Without you, this book would not have been written. I love you dearly! Thank you for all you do!
- I want to acknowledge my five children, Jedediah, Zolani, Elijah, Niara, and Isaac. So much of what I do is with you in mind. When you are old enough to read this book, apply the wisdom therein to your own lives.
- To my parents, Paul and Carrie Grady—Thank you for your unconditional love and support which has given me the passion to help others replicate your example.
- To Pastor Lionel Pointer, Jr. and 1st Lady Dr. Michelle, thank you for raising and nurturing me spiritually. Thank you for modeling

how to love, how to encourage, and how to forgive. Finally, thank you for the prayers.

- To my sister, Janessa—Thank you for your tremendous love and support of me, my family, and the ministry that God has laid on me. Thank you for your labor in editing, your passion for the message, and your encouragement.
- To my brothers Kevin and Paul, thank you for your encouragement, fellowship, and support.
- To my Round Oak Church Family—, thank you for all that you do!
- To the staff at MishaWrites, LLC— thank you Misha and Camille for using your gifts for the Kingdom!
- To my other parents, Jim and Devorah Proctor—thank you for being great parents to me.
- To the countless forerunners that have paved the way for me, thank you!

Contents

Dedication i

Acknowledgments iii

Foreword 1

   I. The Weight of the World. 7

  II. The Empty Place. 21

 III. Woman Behold Thy Daughter. 21

 IV. Sick and Tired. 33

  V. The Road Less Unraveled 39

 VI. A Different Fight. 45

 VII. To Trust or Not to Trust 61

VIII. Fears for Tears. 73

 IX. The Gift that Keeps on Giving. 81

  X. This Woman's Work 91

 XI. The Proof is in the Peace. 103

FOREWORD

THIS BOOK IS dedicated to all the daughters of Mamie, the thousands of women who like me loved and adored their mothers so much that we psychologically walk in and re-possess their shoes long after they are gone. We laugh like they do, cry like they do, love like they do, worship like they do, raise our children like they raised us, and emulate their exact same strength in times of trouble. It's only now that we, the errant daughters, are beginning to see the effects of this perceived inheritance. Truth be told, we're tired, worn, lonely, angry, guilt-ridden, emotionally bankrupt, and hurting simply because we've been walking in someone else's destiny and not our own — for far too long.

Letting go of idols is a difficult process. It is first and foremost a spiritual process because God will cause you to stumble upon things about your idol that can only be revealed and understood in His presence. It seems reverent for me to say to God "I loved my mother." Conversely, I am ashamed to admit to Him "I idolized her." Yet for most of my adult life, I have been trying to emulate my mother and her strength without understanding what it cost her to be so strong. She chose a pathway that most of the time was sorrowful and lonely just to prove to herself and her children that she could take it. It made us look up to her and not to the Source of her strength. She needed that heroic stance because it gave her suffering legitimacy, made all the burdens she had elected to carry seem worthwhile. She could prove at least to her onlookers that she was a survivor. But that's where she stopped. She never heeded the call not just to survive, but to conquer; in fact, to be more than a conqueror. And even before her death, I picked up her gauntlet, and I have been running her fitful race, taking care of everybody and everything around me, except me, ever since.

Understand that my mother was not cruel or willfully negligent in any sense of the word. That's why it's taken so long for me to diagnose or acknowledge her impact on my life. Though sometimes sparse, I always had a warm meal, a roof over my head, and hand-me-down clothes. She made sure I went to school and to church and she disciplined me for the slightest infraction. By most standards, she was an adequate if not good parent. But while she made provisions for most of my physical needs, she neglected my emotional ones. I was a "reconciliation baby," the by-product of one of several reunions between her and my alleged father. Truth is, by the time I was born, she was too exhausted to tend to me because trying to keep up with her husband had zapped all her strength. Thus, the things that would strengthen and nurture a young girl emotionally — like love, gentleness, tenderness, healthy intimacy — were never part of my upbringing. I emerged almost from the womb doomed for emotional failure, and it's been a rough road to tow ever since. This failure manifests itself especially in relationships with men, whether they are my lovers or my sons. I may be there physically, but I am rarely there emotionally.

Not long ago, I had to make a difficult choice. Through a very trying test involving my youngest son, God brought me to the place where I had to acknowledge that Mamie's shoes no longer fit me. I desperately needed to get to a safe place in Him and in order to do so I had to let go of my mother. If you want to experience the liberation that comes from "casting down every idol," you have to be willing to say to your idol, whoever it is, "No more! I love you, but your destiny is not mine." For me, it was a conscious decision to lay down my need to be right and strong and perfect and in control of everybody and everything so that God could lead me and shepherd me to green pastures and still waters and peace and to people who could truly love and care for me. Today I love my mother even more because she is in her rightful place in my life — not my idol, but the vessel deliberately chosen to bring me to this earth for God's divine purpose. I embrace everything that was good about her — her tenacity, frugality, sense of style and love of orderliness. But I am divorcing myself from her inability to love herself and others unconditionally, from her fear of being vulnerable in front of the people who loved her, and from her stoic belief that love hurts all the time and if you're a good Christian, you just endure it all the way from earth to glory with a smile. And with this renewed sense of purpose, I begin a new journey, in my own shoes.

My journey starts at the altar of forgiveness. I am learning how to forgive my mother for the attitudes, values, and behaviors I have because of the secrets she kept, the tears she shed, the man she married, the burdens she allowed to infiltrate our family, her lack of self esteem, her suffering servant mentality, and her impotent god. I am seeking to forgive her for abandoning her dreams, for dying alone and unhappy, and for leaving me here with so much to learn about her now instead of when she was living. I am letting go of my anger at her for not thinking ahead to the day when I would have children and would want to pour into their lives, and for "holding down the fort" rather than "burning down the fort" of emotional abuse and neglect that has buttressed our family for generations. God knows I long for the day when I am finally at peace with my mother. It'll take work, but I'm worth it.

And so are you. I recently heard a story about monkey hunters in Thailand. It seems monkeys are relatively easy prey because all the trapper has to do is put a piece of food in a box with holes cut in the sides. When the monkey sticks his hand in the box and grabs the food, he is immediately caught. The only way to freedom is to let go of the piece of food so that he can retract his hands through the holes. For those of us living in the shadows of our mothers, we have to let go of the unhealthy ties that bind so that we can freely walk into our destiny.

I pray the Holy Spirit will create a great passion for this assignment within you and that He will comfort and guide you to wholeness and wellness.

Misha
November 20, 2010

PART I
THE DIAGNOSIS

The Weight of the World

Casting all your care on Him, for He careth for you[1]

"I feel better, so much better, since I laid my burdens down"[2]

Darlene came to my office for a family counseling session with her husband and adolescent daughter. She came at the pleading of her husband who hoped to save their marriage. She, on the other hand, came to save their adolescent daughter. Their daughter was defiant, failing in school, and experimenting with marijuana. Yet she was wise enough to know what was going on between her parents. Darlene was through with her husband! She had had enough. She had heard his empty promises many times before. According to Darlene, "If my children were in college, the marriage would be over, so over!" Darlene was bitter because she refused to forgive her husband for fifteen years of irresponsibility. She had already told him that she wanted a divorce… an end to the agony. Her husband Bill wanted to save the marriage, but not for altruistic reasons. He depended on her emotionally, physically, and financially, and needed her to continue carrying the load. He was comfortable and was not ready to exit out of his comfort zone. She was tired and worn like Rosa Parks who refused to give up her seat on that Alabama bus. Darlene had been

---

1   1 Peter 5:7 (King James Version)
2   Glory, Glory, Hallelujah/Since I laid my Burdens Down

carrying the weight of her defiant daughter, the weight of her autistic son, the weight of her father who lived with her, and the weight of her needy husband. Most importantly, she had been carrying the heaviest weight of all—— unforgiveness.

It became clear fairly quickly what the source of the problem was in this family. The daughter's defiance was a strategic cry for help, and the husband's desperate request for counseling was his last ditch effort to remain a child. Furthermore, Darlene's disposition, a mix of anger, regret, resentment, worry, and fatigue described the reality of many Black women who carry the weight of the world on their shoulders. She said, "I am so tired of planning everything, doing everything, handling everything." You would have thought my response as a compassionate counselor would have been empathic or sympathetic at a minimum. Instead, my response was, "Well, that's what you wanted. The reason why you married him was because you knew he would not challenge your desire to be in control. You knew he would just go with the flow. But now you are tired and worn. You were not meant to carry this load and now you are beginning to faint." Her face dropped in amazement. Darlene was amazed at the juxtaposition between the audacity and the accuracy of my response. Her expression said it all. It said, "You got me, Doc."

It is no secret that women are stronger than men in many respects. After witnessing my wife endure several pregnancies to deliver five healthy children, I became convinced. If truth were to be told, I have been convinced for a long time that Black women are stronger than Black men in many respects. It is one thing to have a baby in your womb. It is another to have one baby in your womb, one baby on your breast, a toddler on your lap, and what I call, "the weight of the world on your shoulders." I see routinely and remarkably, Black women carrying the load no matter how heavy it is. We have historical examples such as Harriet Tubman carrying the burden of freedom, Rosa Parks carrying the burden of equality, Coretta Scott King carrying the burden of a limitless movement, and we have the Virgin Mary carrying the Burden-Bearer. We have current examples such as Michelle Obama carrying the burden of history in the making, and Oprah carrying the burden of Black entrepreneurship, and Shirley Caesar carrying the burden of gospel music. Then we have current, less famous examples, such as yourself—the one who is reading this book.

Your burdens may be private, but they are nonetheless very heavy. You may be carrying the burden of single-motherhood, the burden of domestic violence, the burden of being sexually abused, the burden of sexual confusion, the burden of abandonment, the burden of failed relationships, the burden of addiction, the burden of divorce, the burden of fatherlessness, the burden of under-appreciation, sickness, loneliness, and the list goes on and on.

While some Black women are coping with one or two of the aforementioned burdens, many are currently dealing or have dealt with many, if not most, of those burdens. I wrote my master's thesis on *Stressful Life Events and Violence as Predictors of Depression in Urban African- American Women*. You are probably wondering why a man would be led to study depression and stress in women. You are theorizing, "Maybe his mother was depressed, or his sister or another loved one." The answer is simple, I was led. I believe the Holy Spirit had ordered my steps accordingly. During my first year in graduate school for clinical psychology, I was assigned an advisor who specialized in working with children. My focus, however, was not on children, but on adults. I was in the adult track of the program, but was assigned to a professor who specialized in children. In terms of research on adults, the only data that was available was the data on the mothers of the children in the research studies. That course of study is where I grew to appreciate the strength of Black women. I had models of strong Black women in my family in the persons of my mother, grandmother, aunts, sister, cousins, and others. Now I had an opportunity to look at the plight more objectively.

One of the measures that I used in my research was a Life Events Scale. It listed several different stressful life events including having an abortion, losing a job, getting divorced, and having a family member who committed suicide. Each woman had to identify the life event she experienced, and then identify the corresponding subjective severity of stress. I found that many women had experienced a cluster of stressful life events which we refer to as cumulative stressful life events. As I began to study this realistic plight of many Black women, the research begged one question in me, "How are these women still alive and functioning well?" The measure of how much weight those women had been, and still are, carrying on their shoulders is mind-boggling. However, this mind-boggling phenomenon led to another question that I had to ask myself: "If many of these women experience the same number and severity of stressors, why are some depressed and not functioning well, while others are doing well despite their ordeal?"

I began to understand why some women become depressed and seemingly can not handle the weight that they are carrying. As the stressors accumulate on the shoulders of women, day by day, week by week, month by month, and year by year, the accumulation of weight overtaxes their natural capacity to function. Similarly, people who are obese have more pressure on their heart, lungs, skin, knees, and back than they can handle. These parts of the body start shutting down, buckling under the excess weight, followed by the onset of weight-related diseases such as heart disease, diabetes, and kidney failure. Well, this principle is also evidenced in emotional obesity. The more emotional weight we accumulate, the more pressure we place on our souls and our bodies to keep the pain at bay. The reality is that many, if not most women are carrying too many emotionally crippling burdens. Indeed, most of the burdens that women carry are unresolved hurts and pains. A burden starts off as a pain that can be healed if attended to. Instead of attending to the pain in its infancy, however, many women avoid the pain until the pain becomes unbearable. It becomes unbearable because the longer the wound goes untreated, the more susceptible to infection it becomes. Specifically, as it relates to hurts and pains, when untreated, a small hurt can progress and manifest into malice. This progression of hurt and pain is illuminated in the chart on the next page.

The Progression of Unresolved Pain

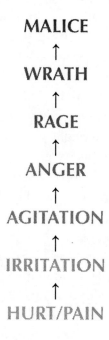

MALICE

↑

WRATH

↑

RAGE

↑

ANGER

↑

AGITATION

↑

IRRITATION

↑

HURT/PAIN

As a person progresses from one stage to another, the intensity of the pain gets stronger and stronger and more and more harmful. The stages always start with hurt/pain. When someone says something or does something that angers you, you feel hurt before you ever feel anger. If you do not acknowledge and express the hurt, it progresses into irritation. If you do not process the irritation, it progresses into agitation. The progression continues from agitation to anger, anger to rage, rage to wrath, and from wrath to malice.

Malice is the desire to harm others or to see others suffer by extreme ill will or spite. Because malice is not socially acceptable, we suppress the emotion to minimize the external manifestation or to prevent an explosive outburst. While you are consciously trying to avoid killing someone else, you are literally slowly killing yourself. Just one occurrence of hurt can cause this. So just imagine if internally 1,000 of these processes are occurring simultaneously. In other words, many women have 20 to 40 years (or more) of unresolved hurts and pain progressing into negative and harmful weight. Just as the force of a volcano erupting is extremely powerful; the energy within you is as powerful. Instead of being an eruption or an explosion, it is an implosion, *meaning you explode internally.*

While you may be overweight physically, emotionally you may be obese. Unless you lose this weight, you will die sooner than you think. Yes, it is a matter of life and death. Heretofore it seems that you have coped with many burdens handily. The weight of the world, however, is getting heavier and heavier. The soul was not meant to carry so much weight. Diseases such as depression, alcoholism, drug addiction, and Post Traumatic Stress Disorder (PTSD) are slowly collapsing the souls of many Black women. In fact, the number one killer of American women is heart disease, and Black women are 35% more likely than Non-Hispanic Americans to die from heart disease.[3]

The overburdened mind is analogous to a computer that is overloaded with files and viruses impacting the available memory. The computer slowly decreases in performance and then ultimately crashes. I see and hear Black women who have been weathering storm after storm, coping with trauma after trauma, and fighting battle after battle get to a place where they say, "I am so tired!" They try to slow down and regroup, but the weight of the world will not let them. Instead, they speed toward an inevitable crash. This decision is a form of suicide. During one of the last scenes in the movie, "Set It Off" starring Jada Pinkett and Queen Latifah, the latter's character, "Cleo," feels that she has no other choice than to drive to her death. She is surrounded by cops and so she feels there is no way out.

However, there is always a way out. The Bible says in 1 Corinthians 10:13, *"There hath no temptation taken you but such as is common to man: but God is faithful, who will not suffer you to be tempted*

---

3   U.S. Department of Heath & Human Services (2007)

above that ye are able; but will with the temptation also make a way of escape that you may be able to bear it."[4] What Queen Latifah's character could and should have done is get to the place of surrender. She would not have escaped from the police, but she still would be alive with the hope of a better life. You may not see how your life is going to change, but I am sure you can admit that if you keep heading in the same direction at the same speed, you will definitely crash.

Take a minute to assess the weight that is on your shoulders. Can you really handle the pressure? Terry Joseph, a character on the cable television series "Soul Food," was an African American woman who thought she could handle the weight. She was a driven, independent, successful lawyer who seemingly could juggle the pressures of life. From the outside it looked like she had it all together. However, after two divorces, other failed relationships, and tremendous pressures at work, she developed a psychological disorder called Panic Disorder where she suffered frequent panic attacks. There will come a point in your life where either you will lose the weight or the weight of the world will crush you. Which outcome do you choose?

---

4   King James Version

Consider all of the weights that are pressing you down. List them and also write their impact on your life. Impact will be measured on a scale of 1-10. A score of 1 means that the weight caused (or is causing) minimal adversity in your life. A score of 10 means the weight caused (or is causing) major adversity in your life.

Weight	Impact Score

The Empty Place

"Like the woman at the well I was seeking for things that could not satisfy."[5]

She is empty, and void, and waste: and the heart melteth, and the knees smite together, and much pain is in all loins, and the faces of them all gather blackness.[6]

SHEILA IS OBESE not just because she eats too much food or rarely exercises. She also is obese because she has let pounds of emotional weight accumulate. Sheila is an emotional eater. She does not eat to live, she lives to eat. Eating seemingly gives her the comfort, nurturance, and understanding that most of the people in her life either cannot or will not give her. She has a special relationship with food and she has tried many diets before, but to no avail. It is not that she has not lost any weight before; she just gains it back—plus some. Sheila feels ashamed, guilty, and most of all, unattractive. Her three best friends are mashed potatoes, cookies and cream ice cream, and quarter-pound cheeseburgers. Sheila's relationship with food began when she was a little girl. She was an introverted child who played by herself most of the time. She had few friends and her parents rarely validated her. She was a pretty girl, but her parents almost never told

---

5   Fill My Cup, Lord/Richard Blanchard
6   Nahum 2:10 (King James Version)

her she was pretty; hence, she developed a poor self image. She also experienced neglect and rarely received attention from her mother. Despite this reality for Sheila, food seemed to always help her to feel better. So naturally, as Sheila grew up and began navigating through the storms of life, food was right there to help her to make it through.

Cognitively, Sheila knows she is an emotional eater and needs to stop. Emotionally, everyone else has forsaken her except for food. How can she abandon the one friend that has stuck with her through thick and thin? Yet, despite her close relationship with food, Sheila feels empty and alone on the inside. Just as she has consumed a great deal of empty calories (foods that fill you up quickly but have little to no meaningful nutrition), Sheila has come to a place in her life where it seems she has nothing to show for her efforts. Like the prodigal son, this prodigal daughter had spent years partying with friends, going to party after party and club after club. However, now when she travels, she travels by herself because all of her friends are gone. Like the woman at the well, Sheila had experienced many relationships. She had been married two times, divorced two times, and dated several other men. The part-time man she is now with is married, just not to her. The blessings that emanated from her relationships with those men are the three children whom she loves. The problem, however, is she continues to put everyone and everything above them; such as partying, romantic relationships, sleep, and television. She knows she has to sacrifice for them and give them more of herself, but she is depleted. She is fatigued. She is empty.

One day, Sheila came into my office with that look of fatigue. Fatigue to anybody else is just fatigue. To Black women, fatigue may be a code name for depression. Many of you reading this book, have either left this place in the text, are pondering the next trip, or have just checked in to what I call "The Empty Place Hotel." I call it this for two reasons. First, you have to pay to stay at the hotel. But the cost is not paid in money, it is paid in time. The longer you stay there, the more time you waste on a life that is unprofitable and unhappy.

Second, there is emptiness there. Checking in to this hotel includes a trip down memory lane where regret, disappointment, and lack of satisfaction fester. Depression also resides at this empty place, which is why so many Black women try to avoid this place like the plague. This avoidance is demonstrated by being busy enough and distracted enough with other matters to avoid focusing on one's own emptiness. However, when you get to the point that no distraction is salient enough to neutralize the deep pain that you feel, you have checked in to your *empty place*.

The "woman at the well" is a woman who travelled to this empty place. She came by herself with an empty vessel while being a mostly empty vessel. She was not completely empty, for she was full of bad memories, disappointments, and regrets. She had her fill of relationships, yet she had nothing good to show for them. Jesus points out that the man she was living with was not even her own man. I see it all the time and it breaks my heart. Many women go from job to job, relationship to relationship, thrill to thrill looking to be filled with something meaningful. No matter how long they dance at the club, no matter how long they work at their jobs, or even how much time they spend at church, many women find themselves at this lonely, insecure, and empty place. Most of the women that I see in my private practice are strong-willed, brilliant, resilient, tenacious, and yet *broken*. And because of the fracture, there is a leak somewhere within the soul that is causing a slow seepage of virtue, of joy, of peace, and of fulfillment. We can assume that the woman at the well was independent, for she went to the well by herself. It is plausible that she was aesthetically appealing because she had many men in her past. No doubt the woman at the well was religious for she not only told Jesus the worship routine of the Samaritans, but she also had enough sense to perceive Him to be a prophet. Nonetheless, even with the aforementioned positive characteristics in her repertoire, she had arrived at her empty place.

If you are at your empty place, neither your looks, your education, your financial stability, nor your determination can sustain you.

Many women believe that temporary gratifications enable them to leave their empty places. However, if you always seem to return to the place that is so miserable, then my question is, "Did you really ever leave?" The water at the well is a metaphor for temporary fulfillment or gratification. The water seemed to quench her thirst, but only temporarily. She had to keep coming back over and over again. So when Jesus painted the picture of a type of water that would quench her thirst once and for all, and cause her never to return to that empty place, she became all ears. After her encounter with the Master, guess what? She left her empty place and she departed the well with joy.

If you are in this place, I have good news for you. Now, before you get pessimistic, let me set the record straight. I am not going to present to you seven secrets to success, the five foundations of favor, nor the three thoughts of thriving. I am not about to provide self-help strategies because the truth is you cannot help yourself. If you could, you would not still be in your empty place. I am also not going to present to you a way to only feel gratified, but I want to share a way for you to be satisfied. There is a profound difference between being gratified and being satisfied. The deceiving attribute about being gratified is that when you are in the height or the apex of your gratification, it feels like real satisfaction. When you use drugs and you are "nice" or "high as a kite," you feel satisfied at that moment. When you go to your favorite shopping mall and get gorgeous outfits for half the price, what a high! When you are at the height of your orgasmic experience, you feel like you are satisfied. When you accomplish that goal or that victory you have worked so hard for, you feel satisfied. It is only when the moment is over do you come to grips with the reality that you really weren't satisfied, but only gratified. When the high wears off, and the orgasm is over, and the world no longer cares about your past accomplishments, you come back to that empty place called temporary gratification, which is depressing. It is analogous to living paycheck to paycheck. You have no wealth stored up to sustain you during hard economic times, and so you survive until the next paycheck. Similarly, because joy, love, and peace are not activated in your life, which will sustain you even during the storms, you live from good time to good time. Are you the one that says, "If I can just make it to the weekend, I can party my sorrows away?" Incidentally, there are women that believe that church is the answer to their empty problem. Not so! I have seen in the past, and continue to see, many empty people at church. Don't get me wrong, the church is a good place to be empty, but only if you are coming to be filled with something powerful. I see many women come to the church empty and leave empty. Either something is wrong with the church, or something is wrong with the empty vessel. I have discovered that most of the time it is not the church it is the vessel. The Apostle Paul in his letter to the church at Ephesus commanded the church to be filled with the Spirit.[7] This command in the Greek literally means *be always being filled with the Spirit*. It refers to a day by day, moment by moment, thought by thought filling. It is not a one time filling, but rather a continual process of allowing the Holy Spirit to rule your soul. When you allow the Holy Spirit to rule your soul (mind, will, emotions), the first order of business is to purge you of thoughts and tendencies that don't give GOD any glory. The problem with many women even at church is that their lives are filled with empty experiences, fears, doubts, lusts, and patterns of thinking that are contrary to the will of GOD. The solution, therefore, is to allow the Holy Spirit to take you to a real empty place by purging and purifying you. Psalms 51 is one of the most humble and surrendering prayers in the Bible. In verses 7 and 8, David says, *"Purge me with hyssop, and I shall be clean: wash me, and I shall be whiter than snow. Make me to hear joy and gladness; that the bones which thou hast broken may rejoice.[8]* I recommend praying a prayer similar to the above prayer, but making it personal to your empty place. After you arrive at this empty place, you can allow yourself to be filled with the Holy Spirit.

---

7   Ephesians 5:18 (King James Version)
8   King James Bible

Describe the people, places, and things that you thought would sat-isfy you, but only provided temporary gratification. Describe how empty you really felt.

_____

_____

_____

_____

_____

_____

_____

_____

_____

_____

_____

_____

_____

_____

_____

_____

_____

_____

_____

_____

_____

_____

Woman, Behold Thy Daughter

For I acknowledge my transgressions [9]

"We'll walk hand and hand some day" [10]

LAUREN CAME TO my office for counseling because her son was having behavioral problems. Soon into the interview I realized that Lauren needed counseling as well. She wasn't "crazy," but she carried a great deal of pain. During her individual sessions, Lauren would cry easily as she mentioned the multitude of stressors in her life. She indeed has major stress in her life; however, everywhere Lauren went, it seemed stress either followed her there or was already there when she arrived. She was attracted to the same type of man, and she tried to medicate her pain with marijuana and sex. She had four children, all with four different men. You are probably wondering about the type of relationship she had with her father. You are probably hypothesizing that her relationship with her father is the major cause for her current behavior and emotional state. Well, it is true that she did not have a good relationship with her father. What is more profound than the relationship between a daughter and her father, however, is the relationship between a daughter and her mother. When I began to ask questions about her relationship with her mother, Lauren initially

---

9   Psalms 51:3 (King James Version)
10   We Shall Overcome

responded sternly that their relationship was strained. As she began to describe her childhood, I realized that she questioned whether her mother really loved her. I asked, "Did your mother love you?" She responded quickly and decisively, "Of course she loved me. I know she loved me. She took care of me." Immediately her countenance began to change and went into deep thought. Her facial expression communicated that she questioned the sincerity of her mother's love. The notion that your mother doesn't love you is just too much to handle for most people. It is the type of pain that seems to hurt in a place that nobody, even God, can get to. At least it seems that way sometimes. I knew that Lauren's mother probably tried to love her, but to Lauren it probably didn't feel like love. Hence, I asked Lauren, "Did it feel like your mother loved you?" She immediately responded "No," which led me to ask this philosophical but relevant question, "Is love really love if you can't feel it?"

Speaking of love, one of Jesus' final statements when he was on the cross was a compelling command. He said, *"Woman, behold thy son."*[11] Referring to John, his beloved disciple, Jesus, even while dying, understood the mother's need to mother, and the need of every human being to be mothered. That word *behold* in the Greek means literally "lo" or "see" and it is used as an imperative. Jesus was in a sense saying to Mary, take advantage of this opportunity to be a mother to John. For the purposes of this book, I am encouraging mothers to behold their daughters and daughters to behold their mothers. My expectation of readers of this chapter specifically, and this book in general, is to "see" the dynamics of what is really going on. I am reminded of the popular phrase, "Mothers love their sons and raise their daughters." In my experience as a psychologist, as a counseling minister, and as someone who spends considerable time helping families, that phrase applies to many African American mothers and daughters. Many Black daughters are in counseling, psychotherapy, rehabilitation, and in states of depression due to a lifelong legitimate belief that their mothers didn't love them. The reality is that many of

---

11   John 19:26 King James Version

these mothers really do, in fact, attempt to love their daughters, but their love is misunderstood and hidden in toughness, verbal abuse, and lack of nurturing. Now, let me be clear, not every mother loves her daughter. There are many women who become pregnant and subsequently, while the child is in the womb and thereafter, refuse to love, nurture, and protect their child. I am not referring to those mothers. I am referring to mothers who raise their daughters to be independent; mothers who rarely nurture their daughters with words or hugs and often criticize their daughters; mothers who throw guilt trips on their daughters; and mothers who belittle their daughter's father.

If you fit the above description of the mother who attempts to love her daughter, but the application of that love seems to be contradictory, it is time to behold thy daughter. We need to examine how to behold thy daughter; however, first we need to explore where this relational tendency possessed by many African American mothers comes from. Let's take a look at parenting practices in slave times.

There are many dynamics between African mothers and daughters that occurred before the Trans-Atlantic Slave Trade. However, the tendencies that were established during American slavery give greater insight into the current dynamic between Black mothers and daughters in America. This dynamic is actually described in detail in the Willie Lynch speech entitled, *"How To Make a Slave."*[12] The portion of the speech which is germane to this chapter appears below.

THE BREAKING PROCESS OF THE AFRICAN WOMAN

Take the female and run a series of tests on her to see if she will submit to your desires willingly. Test her in every way, because she is the most important factor for good economics. If she shows any sign of resistance in submitting completely to your will, do not hesitate to use the bull whip on her to extract that last bit of b-word out of her. Take care not to kill her, for in doing so, you spoil good economics. When in complete submission, she will train her off springs in the

---

12   Speech delivered by Willie Lynch in 1712

early years to submit to labor when she becomes of age. Un-
derstanding is the best thing. Therefore, we shall go deeper
into this area of the subject matter concerning what we have
produced here in this breaking process of the female Nigger.
We have reversed the relationship. In her natural uncivilized
state she would have a strong dependency on the uncivilized
Nigger male, and she would have a limited protective tenden-
cy toward her independent male offspring and would raise
male off springs to be dependent like her. Nature had pro-
vided for this type of balance. We reversed nature by burning
and pulling a civilized Nigger apart and bull whipping the
other to the point of death, all in her presence. By her being
left alone, unprotected, with the MALE IMAGE DESTROYED,
the ordeal caused her to move from her psychological de-
pendent state to a frozen independent state. In this frozen
psychological state of independence, she will raise her MALE
and female offspring in reversed roles. For FEAR of the young
males life she will psychologically train him to be MENTALLY
WEAK and DEPENDENT, but PHYSICALLY STRONG. Because
she has become psychologically independent, she will train
her FEMALE off springs to be psychologically independent.
What have you got? You've got the Nigger WOMAN OUT
FRONT AND THE OLD MAN BEHIND AND SCARED. This is
a perfect situation of sound sleep and economics. Before the
breaking process, we had to be alertly on guard at all times.
Now we can sleep soundly, for out of frozen fear his woman
stands guard for us. He cannot get past her early slave mold-
ing process. He is a good tool, now ready to be tied to the
horse at a tender age. By the time a Nigger boy reaches the
age of sixteen, he is soundly broken in and ready for a long life
of sound and efficient work and the reproduction of a unit of
good labor force. Continually through the breaking of the un-
civilized savage Nigger, by throwing the Nigger female savage
into a frozen psychological state of independence, by killing

off the protective male image, and by creating a submissive dependent mind of the Nigger male slave, we have created an orbiting cycle that turns on its own axis forever, unless a phenomenon occurs and re shifts the position of the male and female slaves.

Willie Lynch was considered an expert in developing, maintaining, and getting the most out of slaves. In fact, he bragged on his plan positing that the fruits of the principles he espoused could last hundreds of years, even forever. Under the heading of "reversing nature," he taught that Black mothers should raise their sons to be physically strong, yet mentally and psychologically dependent on them. On the other hand, he taught that Black mothers should raise their daughters to be mentally and psychologically independent. This was a reversal in nature because even though many African cultures were matriarchal and matrilineal, the men were still considered the leaders of the families. This leadership included providing for, protecting, and carrying the weight of the families on their shoulders. One of the tactics that Willie Lynch taught, was to separate the husband from the wife. When the wife was attacked, whipped, raped, and disrespected, the husband instinctually would come back and do anything and everything in his power to protect his wife and family. The purposeful consequence for Black men who attempted to protect their family would be public hanging and castration. (Now, some of you who are reading this are wrongly assuming that I am blaming the "White Man" or slavery for the current condition. On the contrary, I am providing insight into historical events which led to this specific and unique type of parenting behavior. This discussion is a cornerstone for mothers to assume responsibility for incomplete parenting.)

Now, the public hanging and castration was designed to instill an intense fear in the mind of the mother. In other words, the mother had to move into survival mode. In her psyche, the mother was thinking that *if I raise my son to be mentally strong and psychologically independent, then he will end up just like my husband…dead! Hence, for him to survive, I need to raise my son to be dependent on me, and my daughter to be independent. If he is dependent on me, I will be able to protect him. My daughter will be strong enough to take care of herself.*

Lest you think I am going to criticize this decision, actually, let me quickly state that actually it was the best decision those slave mothers could have made at the time. Even though this was a plan designed by the enemy, God can take the evil and work it out for our good. Because of that survival-based decision, we continue to have strong Black women who survive and thrive as the single heads of their households and function in many different roles. Due to the traumas of slavery, the intense warfare of racism, and the failure of many Black men to assume responsibility for our families and communities, African Americans as a race have survived largely because of the grace that God has given to African American women. When you are in a war, the best way to win the war is to stay alive. The choice to raise black men to be dependent on their mother was a decision of survival.

Today, hundreds of years later, we see the impact of that decision. The decision should have been a temporary solution; one hundred years after slavery was abolished, we should have regrouped. But the ramifications are compelling. We have grown men in their forties, fifties and even sixties living at home with or financially dependent on their mothers. We have Black men who date, sleep with, pursue, and even marry women who will take care of them. Sugar mommas are the new sugar daddies! And, for the purposes of this book, we have daughters who were raised not to depend on a man, but to be tough and resilient, no matter the pain, the trauma and the hurt, and without ever changing the stern poker face. In T.D. Jakes' movie, *"Woman, Thou Art Loosed,"* Bishop Jakes is preaching a revival and accurately says, "We live in a get over it generation. Everybody wants you to get over it." Many African American mothers teach their daughters to "get over it" without the comfort, the guidance, and the compassion needed to do so. Generations of women enter into abusive, exploitive, and unfulfilling relationships because their mothers haven't allowed themselves to be healed. Once this healing occurs, however, it now becomes possible to not only love their daughters unconditionally, but to share with them experiential wisdom. You cannot teach what you have not learned.

Mothers, you have great insight into the pain of your daughters due to the intensity of your own pain. You are/were a daughter of a mother caught up in this cycle. You know how it feels. You say, "Well, that's how I was raised, and look how I turned out. I am intelligent, wealthy, and independent." The adjective that is most frequently left out though is happy or whole. You know what it's like to long for your mother's affection, nurturance, validation, approval, warmth, and love and you wonder, "Will I ever experience it?" Well, what is the solution? Mothers, you need to forgive your mothers (deceased or still living) in order to have the capacity to behold your daughters. If your mother was human, then she was not perfect and definitely made some mistakes. Some of these mistakes were extremely painful to you. There are some mothers who refuse to believe that their boyfriend molested their daughter. There are some mothers whose daughter reminds them of themselves, which for some is unbearable. Some mothers physically and verbally abused their daughters. Some mothers never really understood their daughters. But, as discussed in the three steps below, it is not too late to behold your daughter.

1) Awareness

Awareness is the first step. Before change can occur, there must be awareness that change needs to occur. One has to admit that there is a problem. The mantra has been, "This is how I was raised" or "Look at how I turned out." If that was your argument and I was opposing counsel, I would say, "I rest my case, Your Honor!" No matter how hard you try to mask or forget the pain of your relationship with your mother, the evidence of its ill effects is overwhelming. The reality is that awareness is a humbling experience. It forces you to deal with who you really are and not who you wish you were. Likewise, one cannot be saved until the sinner is *aware* of his/her sinfulness and comes to the realization that he/she needs a savior. If you did not think or were aware that you were a sinner, you would not need a savior.

This notion of awareness is two-fold. Not only do you have to be aware of your relationship with your mother, but you also have to be aware of the fact that you have recycled the same parenting style with your own daughter. In other words, the same void that is in you is the same void that is in your daughter. The reality is that there are blind spots that prevent us from really seeing what we need to see. When you look out of your driver side mirror, it is virtually impossible to see a car that is next to you. Because you don't see any cars, you may attempt to switch lanes which may cause an accident. You were looking in the right place, but you did not see what you needed to see. I believe that many mothers do look in the right places; however, the blind spots prevent them from seeing and understanding that the same parenting style that hurt them as children is the same style they use with their own daughters. Not only must the mothers be aware, but the daughters also must be aware. I am placing the emphasis on mothers to behold their daughters; however, it is still the responsibility of daughters to behold their mothers even if their mothers do not behold them.

2) Articulation

After you become aware that this dynamic exists in your relationship with your mother and/or daughter(s), you must articulate the hurt and pain in its original and raw state.

When people have a great deal of unresolved pain, they usually describe their pain and disappointments in terms of being angry, irritated, or frustrated. If you felt abandoned by your mother, you need to articulate the feeling as being abandoned or as being rejected. Articulation forces you to pinpoint the exact feelings, which is an important component in the process of forgiveness. I have had many clients whom I have counseled to articulate that their mothers really did not love them. They said, "I want to believe that she loved me, but it did not feel like she did." Articulation forces the individual to step outside of denial and other defense mechanisms such as rationalization and projection, and deal with reality. This reality is a painful reality, but articulation sheds light on the root of the problem in order for it to be resolved. In Mark 5:9, Jesus asked for the unclean spirit's name. Many people desperately want to be healed, but they don't want to name the demons that are responsible for keeping them sick. Articulation pinpoints the brutal truth which forces resolution. Many families are dysfunctional because of family secrets still lurking in the closets. There are generations of molestation, incest, rape, addiction, adultery, abuse and other demons that persist in families because the members in the family have been hushed to secrecy. It is the responsibility of the one who is hurt to articulate the damage that was done. The sincere, unfeigned love and affection that mothers and daughters need to have for each other will only occur if one is successfully aware of the problem, and then articulates the nature of the problem. After articulation, the last step toward healing is the expression of affection.

3) Affection

Jesus' declaration on the cross, "*Woman, Behold thy son,*"[13] was the word of *affection*. His words demonstrated the affection that he had for his mother. Smiles are good, genuine hugs are wonderful, but sincere words of encouragement are priceless. Proverbs 18:21 says, "*Death and life are in the power of the tongue.*"[14] Once you have become aware of this dynamic, have articulated your own hurts and have healed, it is time to infuse your daughter(s) with life-giving words. The words, "I apologize" or "I am sorry" are very important. It has been said that, "love means never having to say I'm sorry." While

13   John 19:26 (King James Version)
14   King James Version

your ability to forgive should not be conditioned on hearing the magic words, "I am sorry," your ability to reconcile those you have hurt will be stymied if you yourself won't utter these words and actually mean them. Also, words of affection such as "I love you," and "I am proud of you," and "you are beautiful" are indispensable in providing refreshment to thirsty souls. Giving hugs is another way of expressing affection and communicating emotional closeness. With affection, you have the power to "affect" one's life.

According to a National Institutes of Health (NIH) study,[15] at the center of how our bodies respond to love and affection is a hormone called oxytocin. Most of our oxytocin is made in the area of the brain called the hypothalamus. Some of this hormone is released into our bloodstream, but much of its effect is hypothesized to reside in the brain. Oxytocin makes us feel good when we are close to family and other loved ones. It does this by acting through what scientists call the dopamine reward system. Dopamine is a brain chemical that plays a crucial part in how we perceive pleasure. Problems with the dopamine reward system can lead to serious depression and other mental illnesses.

Oxytocin does more than make us feel good. It lowers the levels of stress hormones in the body, reducing blood pressure, improving mood, increasing tolerance for pain and perhaps even speeding how fast wounds heal. It also seems to play an important role in our relationships. It has been linked, for example, to how much we trust others. The study goes on to say that the same holds true for mothers and infants: they both produce higher levels of oxytocin when they have lots of warm contact with each other.

Unfortunately, the survival formula that many African American mothers were raised on was the notion that if you are tough, cold, and not nurturing to your daughters, they will become independent and successful, which is the main thesis of Willie Lynch. The truth of the matter is that, with sincere affection, your daughters can be raised to be independent, dependent, and also interdependent. God's formula

---

15   NIH Study, "*The Power of Love*", Feb. 2007

for reconciliation assures us that it is never too late. While you and your daughter are still alive, *behold thy daughter*! Likewise, daughter, it is imperative that you behold and forgive your mother. Your mother may have smoked crack and drank alcohol while pregnant with you; she may have abandoned and neglected you; she may have physically, emotionally, or verbally abused you, and blamed you for you being sexually abused. Your mother may not have shared with you experiential wisdom so you could avoid the traps that ensnared her. Whatever mistakes your mother made, it did not catch GOD by surprise. HE permitted whatever pain for your growth and for HIS glory. Furthermore, GOD has empowered you with the ability to forgive, if you are willing.

Mothers: Describe the mistakes you have made with your children (sons and daughters). Have you confessed your mistakes and apologized? Are there family secrets you have yet to share with your children? Are there secrets for which you have sworn your daughter to secrecy?

_____

_____

_____

_____

_____

_____

_____

_____

_____

_____

_____

_____

Daughters: Describe the experiences with your mother or the maternal influence that raised you. Are there hurts and pains deep down that have not been resolved? Have you fully forgiven her for her mistakes?

_____

_____

_____

_____

_____

_____

_____

_____

_____

_____

_____

_____

_____

_____

_____

_____

_____

_____

_____

_____

_____

_____

_____

Sick and Tired

"For this cause many are weak and sickly among you, and many sleep."[16]

DONNETTA ARRIVED AT her counseling session noticeably agitated. Some women have the uncanny ability to mask their unraveling emotional state with a poker face. Not Donnetta! Agitation oozed out of her disposition as if she were looking for a fight. When she looked at me, I felt as if I was her opponent.

It is my therapeutic custom when I begin my counseling sessions to ask clients for good news. My rationale is two-fold. First, life is never all bad. There is always something that is good in your life. Second, the wisdom in Philippians 4:8 instructs us to think on the things that are true, honest, just, pure, lovely, and of a good report. Again, the psychological data proves that the action urged by that verse is emotionally, and physiologically restorative.

Donnetta, with her hands folded, her defiance well-rooted, and her attitude revved up, looked at me and said, "I don't have no good news." She had the ability to speak proper English, but her double negative was born out of frustration. At great length she proceeded to talk about all of the bad things in her life. She mentioned having problems with her children, her job, her husband, her co-workers, church members, life, and even God. She identified emotions symptomatic

---

16   1 Corinthians 11:29-30 (King James Version)

of depression, rage, anxiety, fear, fatigue, hostility, and confusion. Her moods seemed to vacillate between sadness to intense anger. Right before tears met her cheek bone; Donnetta collected herself, wiped her tears, and started complaining again. This went on for twenty minutes. Since this was the initial session, my job was to take the information she shared, and come up with a diagnosis. Her symptoms did not meet the clinical criteria for depression or an anxiety disorder. She was not psychotic nor in the midst of grieving the loss of a loved one. It was not until the end of our session that I finally determined the correct diagnosis for Donnetta. Her diagnosis was that she was *sick and tired of being sick and tired!* Now, you may not find this diagnosis in the psychiatric classification system; nonetheless, many women have symptoms of this diagnosis. Black women, in particular, whether or not they ever go to counseling, will receive this diagnosis some time in their lives. This diagnosis is indeed an idiom and a cliché, but it accurately describes the universal condition of so many Black women. Just ask yourself a question, and even poll your female friends. How many times you have complained about being sick? When I say sick I don't mean physically sick. I mean psychologically sick: sick of the job; sick of the kids; sick of your husband/boyfriend, and if you are honest you or they might say that you are sick of life. Now ask yourself and others around you how many times have they complained about being tired? Tired physically, tired emotionally, tired of not having enough, tired of the lies, tired of doing everything, tired of struggling, and if we are being honest, tired of living.

The reason so many Black women are sick and tired is that their emotions are working overtime, and instead of wellness as the outcome, sickness is the result. Emotions are not just feelings, but rather they are thoughts and perceptions combined with feelings. Specifically, your thinking actually influences your feelings. This is why Philippians 4:8 is so profound. The more time you spend thinking, meditating, and dwelling on something, the more powerful those things become in your immediate reality. Unfortunately, many people focus on negative things which perpetuate fear, doubt, anxiety, depression, anger, etc., things which inhibit healing and, in fact, perpetuate illness. Furthermore, if you have unforgiveness and unresolved hurts and pains on the inside, negative thinking binds to your hurts from the past and further intensifies the sickness and fatigue.

A familiar scripture we read at Communion service is found in 1 Corinthians 11:29-30. It reads, "For he that eateth and drinketh unworthily, eateth and drinketh damnation to himself, not discerning the Lord's body. For this cause many are weak and sickly among you, and many sleep." In verse 28, the Apostle Paul encourages prospective partakers of Communion to examine themselves. When you go to the doctor for a check-up, he/she usually performs an examination to assess what and where the problems are. In the Corinthian church, during the time of the scripture, many people used the elements (bread and wine) for carnal purposes (hunger) and not for spiritual purposes (continued healing). In essence, they neglected the true meaning and value of the ordinance. The ramifications of this practice included judgment resulting in sickness and death. Now, here is the parallel. Many Black women are sick and tired and they don't have to be. The culprit is the refusal to receive God's grace with faith and activate it for your benefit.

God's grace is activated by your proximity to Him. Nowadays in restaurant bathrooms, they have paper towel machines that are activated by motion sensors. When you come close enough to the machine, it becomes activated and begins dispensing paper towels. That is how God works. Nothing will happen if you stay distant from God. Even though He has a supply and is ready to dispense, He won't dispense until His grace is activated. This means you must, by faith, comes close to Him with an expectant heart. What this means for the "sick and tired" is to exchange your burdens for God's peace, your sickness for His healing, your fatigue for His refreshing. This is really what Communion is supposed to offer. However, for this to happen, every individual must come to the realization that she cannot handle her own burdens. She must realize that the weight of the world is too heavy to bear, and one more burden may collapse her soul.

Are you or were you at the place where you are sick and tired? Describe how you got to that place. What are you doing (did you do) to leave this place?

_____

_____

_____

_____

_____

_____

_____

_____

_____

_____

_____

_____

_____

_____

_____

_____

_____

_____

_____

_____

PART II

THE DILEMMA

The Road Less Unraveled

He leads me in the paths of righteousness for his name's sake.[17]

SAVOY WOKE UP early in the morning excited about her road trip. She enjoyed driving alone because it allowed her to think about things, talk with GOD, and most importantly listen to the music she wanted to listen to. She was headed to a wedding as she was one of the bridesmaids. She had to make tracks, because she woke up later than expected. Savoy lived in Washington, D.C., and the wedding was in Raleigh, North Carolina; hence, she figured she had enough time if she hurried. It was 9am and the wedding started at 3pm. She was supposed to meet the bride and the other bridesmaids at a hotel near the ceremony site. This road trip started off extremely pleasant for Savoy. The weather was beautiful, she had her morning coffee, and Jill Scott's *Golden* was playing on the radio. Traffic seemed light and she predicted that she would arrive sooner than expected. Life felt good and Savoy was in the driver's seat. Soon after the song ended, Savoy got a strong urge to pull out the Mapquest directions. After considering the matter seriously, she decided that she would get to her destination without the instructions. She had driven to Raleigh before, and was pretty confident that she could get to the destination without Mapquest.

---

17   Psalms 23:3 (New King James Version)

The strong urge that Savoy received was the Holy Spirit informing her that she needed to change her course. What Savoy did not realize in her haste was that the Mapquest directions she printed out that morning would take her in a direction she had never travelled. She would usually click the shortest distance icon on Mapquest; however, this time she accidentally clicked the shortest time icon. What she did not know was that her accidentally clicking on a different icon was God working in her to get her to her destination. God knew in advance what was literally down the pike. The strong urge that Savoy received while driving was another attempt by the Holy Spirit to get her to change her course. Well, Savoy got on the highway, and before she knew it she was trapped on the highway because a big truck carrying flammable and corrosive chemicals had crashed and spilled its contents. A major fire ensued and the highway was immediately closed. The morning filled with joyful expectation ended in utter dismay and frustration. Savoy did not make it to North Carolina that day. After moving fifteen miles in 5 hours, Savoy decided to go back home.

Savoy's experience on that day is metaphorical to the journey of many Black women. They "sit down" in the driver's seat endeavoring to arrive at their intended destination, only to find themselves stuck, stagnant, and seething with frustration. The real philosophical question is *why*. Why didn't Savoy make it to the wedding? Why does it seem like many Black women find themselves stuck in the middle of the road. Well, there are two main reasons why Savoy did not make it to her destination. First, she took the wrong path; and, second, she was in the driver's seat. There are two main paths in life: the road that is most travelled and the road that is less unraveled. The former road is a road that makes sense for us to take based on logic and our perceptual reasoning. It seems safer and it seems that it is the simplest way to arrive at our destination. The problem with this path is that there are things that we are unable to see on this path and that will ultimately slow us down and stop us from progressing. The latter path, the path that is less unraveled is the path taken by those who walk by faith. It is a path that God unravels as you travel on it. Here is the thing though: God has to be the driver on this path. He knows where you are going, He knows how to get you there; and most importantly, He knows what he wants you to go through while on this journey. The psalmist reminds us that the *"Lord is my shepherd. He leads me in the paths of righteousness for His name's sake."*[18]

Hence, there is a path that leads to righteousness when led by the Shepherd, and there is a path that leads to destruction when led by us. These two paths can be titled, "coping and healing". Coping is the road that many Black women take, while healing is the path that is less unraveled. The difference between the two is profound. Coping is a subjective process in which the individual decides what type of path she wants to undertake. The individual also decides what will help her make it through. It is important to note that coping can be a very beneficial process, especially after major trauma. After major trauma, the body and mind may not be ready to heal, so there must be a coping process that helps the person survive. Coping, however, should be a temporary process rather than a lifelong process. Black women have utilized their resilience and determination to survive the moment, endure the storm, and make it through the battle. Specifically, they decide to do whatever they have to do to endure. If that means working three jobs, or working full time while going to school and raising a family by themselves, that's what they do. If that means channeling the intense pain of the past into an insatiable drive for success, then that is what they do. If that means going to Sunday service, prayer meeting, and Bible study to get through the week that is what they do. Some Black women neglect themselves and their families by being in church too much; coping under the guise of worship. The above examples are what many would consider to be relatively healthy examples of coping. Unfortunately, many Black women have used unhealthy coping strategies such as drugs, alcohol, promiscuity, and partying to escape their painful reality. Whether the coping is healthy or unhealthy, prolonged coping is a human decision rather

---

18   Psalms 23:1,3(New King James Version)

than a divine decision.

Healing, on the other hand, involves surrendering to a process over which the individual has no control. True healing emanates from God. He is Jehovah Rophe, the Lord Our Healer. In coping, the individual decides how much she can take. She decides whether or not she can be still and allow God to heal her. She decides how much she can bear. In healing, however, the individual must place her trust in God. It is God who decides how much she can bear. It is God who decides the timing and instruments of healing.

Invariably, there will come a point in life where coping yields diminishing returns. The coping resources will be no match for the divine purpose and will of God. Many strong, independent, and successful women come to my office when they have reached the end of their coping. They have travelled miles and miles and miles, but still could not get to their intended destination: joy and peace. They are miles away from joy and peace because they did not take the path of forgiveness. Right before they drive to their own demise, they stop and ask me for directions. I tell them, "Stop and get out of the driver's seat. Get in the passenger's seat, and let the Shepherd start driving." It won't be a smooth ride because you have to go through some mountains and valleys. You don't have to navigate and ask the driver if He knows where He is going. Just be still and allow Him to heal the deep places in your soul. As you travel on this road, the Shepherd will begin to unravel your purpose and your destiny to you. In other words, He will begin to explain to you why you had to go through all of the mess you had to go through. You will understand that He was preparing you for a great work. The final thing that I usually say is, "You will be tempted to jump out of the vehicle based on what you see. Just trust the Shepherd for he will undoubtedly lead you to your destination."

Think about how long you have been in the driver's seat. Describe the wrong turns and situations where you were lost while in the driver's seat.

_____

_____

_____

_____

_____

_____

_____

_____

_____

_____

_____

_____

_____

_____

_____

_____

_____

_____

_____

_____

_____

_____

_____

_____

_____

A Different Fight

"I'm so excited and I just can't hide it. I'm about to lose control and I think I like it."[19]

My grace is sufficient for you, for My strength is made perfect in weakness.[20]

HAVE YOU HEARD the expression, "tough as nails?" Well, this expression describes La Tasha. She is tough, fierce, and driven. She is not big, burly, or muscular. By looking at her build, you would not be able to fathom the enormity of her strength. Her strength and toughness come from inside. She was raised to be tough, but not on purpose. You see, La Tasha raised herself. She felt it was the only way to survive. She had witnessed her father physically, emotionally, and verbally abuse her mother. Not on just one occasion, but this happened repeatedly. As a little girl, she stood there paralyzed. She was confused. Should she protect her mother because deep down she knew her mother did not deserve this? Should she try to comfort her daddy because he seemed so angry? As she got older she began to understand that dad was an abusive alcoholic and that he was literally killing her mother's spirit. While LaTasha did not intervene, she vowed that she would never allow a man to abuse her in any capacity.

---

19   "I'm So Excited (Pointer Sisters)
20   II Corinthians 12:9 (New King James Version)

Ever! Unfortunately, LaTasha has broken her vow. She has married a jealous adulterer who doesn't physically abuse her, but rather verbally and emotionally abuses her, which seems to cut through her soul with a more excruciating pain than the blow of a fist to her face.

In times of honest and painful reflection, she asked herself the familiar question, "How did I get here?" Well, she became her own best friend, depending on her will to navigate the twists and turns of life. Due to this determination and drive, La Tasha became extremely successful. She is successful in her career. She has an uncanny ability to minimize disappointment and channel her energies to accomplish academic and occupational success. While her success seems rewarding, it is nonetheless overshadowed by her difficulties in relationships. Though she is a strong fighter with a warrior spirit, she is getting progressively weaker and fainting seems like the only choice for her. I experience this phenomenon first-hand in my practice. I see strong Black women get to the place where they are tapped out and close to giving up.

The characteristic that has been correlated and interwoven with the resilience of Black women is their strength. This strength is demonstrated in their ability to fight—fight giving up, fight injustice, fight defeat. It is recorded that Harriet Tubman risked death and returned from freedom to slavery over 19 times in order to save her people. With a loaded gun, she demanded freedom from slaves who were afraid to be free. Convincingly, she demanded, *"be free or die."*

The nature of resilience is not a new concept for African American women. When we search the historical accounts which document the brutal, dehumanizing atrocities of the Middle Passage and slavery, we cannot help but marvel at the ability of African Americans in general, and African American women in particular, to rebound from such an experience. An African American woman historian, Marimba Ani, writes:

> *"There is no doubt that the shock of slavery was traumatic for us. The culture from which we had been taken was humanly*

*oriented, organized on the basis of the recognition of the hu-
man need for love, warmth, and interrelationship.[21] Oppressed
by dehumanizing circumstances, we still found something
in which to recognize enough of ourselves to revitalize our
souls—to create new selves."[22]*

What is remarkable about the resilience that many Black women
possess is that they can tap into it at the most unlikely times. The situations and seasons where there face the most opposition, the most
destructive storms, and the least amount of support, are the very times
that this resilience is expressed. I have a tremendous amount of respect for single mothers who do a great job raising their children. My
wife and I have our hands full with our children and there are two of
us. I tried to imagine if there was only her. How would she manage?
The reality is that many single mothers manage against what seem to
be insurmountable odds. I have great respect for women who have
been abused and neglected, but despite their extremely painful experiences are able to have joy and live productive and fruitful lives. You
would think the cycle of abuse and neglect would continue generation after generation, but the remarkable resilience of a woman says,
"The buck stops here."

Resilience is analogous to the concept of contentment. The
Apostle Paul in his letter to the church at Philippi talks about being
content. He says, *"Whatever state I am in, I have learned how to
be content. I know how to be abased, and I know how to abound.
Everywhere and in all things, I have been instructed to be both full
and hungry, to abound and to suffer need."[23]* In the Greek concept,
the word *content* means to be *self-sufficient*. In other words, there is
something on the inside that will rise up to handle any situation or
circumstance. Many African American women have this remarkable
resilience within them, and it is vital that they, on a more consistent
basis, tap into it. In another letter, the Apostle Paul tells Timothy to stir

---

21   Let the Circle Be Unbroken (Page 12)
22   Let The Circle Be Unbroken (Page 14)
23   Philippians 4:11,12 (New King James Version)

up the gift that's within you.[24] This precisely is my directive to Black women. Stir up this remarkable gift that is within you. The truth of the matter is that you should have fainted a long time ago. With all that has happened to you, all the drama, the disappointments, the trauma, and letdowns that have befallen you, you are still standing. That is re-markable! Now, I don't want you to take full credit for the resilience, for it is not all your doing. GOD has placed that spirit inside of you. However, for the spirit to be operational and efficacious within you, you have to be His partner. GOD's strength is made perfect in your weakness.

The ability to be resilient and reach deep down within and mus-ter enough energy to get the job done is remarkable. However, when the supply of resilience is depleted and the will and strength to fight is gone, the fight or the battle is still not over. What needs to change is not the inclination to fight, but the manner in which you fight. While the strong and resilient warrior spirit has brought humanity and people of color in particular a long way, it was not designed to take us to the Promised Land. GOD gave you a measure of strength to get from the point of death to the point of being a survivor. The difficulty with just being a survivor, however, is that there is a possibility of suc-cumbing to that which you have already survived.

For example, there are many cancer survivors who after some years succumb to and eventually die of cancer. As a survivor, they have won the battle, but not the war. GOD wants us to not only be survivors, but he wants us also to become conquerors. As a conqueror, you are now occupying the territory that your enemy once occupied. In the analogy of cancer, the cancer can no longer stay in the cells of the body when you conquer it. It must retreat out of the body. Truth be told, GOD still is not satisfied with you being just a conqueror, for he wants you to be *more* than a conqueror. Being more than a conqueror means you have supremacy over what you have conquered. In other words, the "spiritual or emotional" cancer will have a very difficult time returning, unless by your permission. Even if the cancer does

---

24   II Timothy 1:6 (New King James Version)

come back, it won't have the power to overtake you.

Well, what does being more than a conqueror look like practically? It looks like someone who has been delivered from an addiction. In recovery circles, the mantra is, "once an addict always an addict." I completely disagree with that statement. If I have been delivered from something that used to define me, then I am no longer under the supremacy of that addiction. Hence, being more than a conqueror means that you have been delivered from an addiction. Furthermore, not only have you been delivered from the addiction, but you are no longer tempted by that thing. This deliverance or conquering can only happen with a power that is greater than the addictive agent and the human desire to use that agent. In other words, once you consistently yield to the power that delivered you, you have supremacy over the addiction both now and forever.

Obtaining this supremacy or becoming more than a conqueror depends on who you depend on. The Apostle Paul says in Romans 8:35-36[25], *"Who shall separate us from the love of Christ? Shall tribulation, or distress, or persecution, or famine, or nakedness, or peril, or sword? As it is written, For thy sake we are killed all the day long; we are accounted as sheep for the slaughter."* Then he answers the question in verse 37. He says, *"Nay, in all these things we are more than conquerors through him that loved us."*[26] The key phrase in the aforementioned scripture is "through him." This is the revelation I want you to get. Since being more than a conqueror is only achieved through Jesus, the battle or the fight is not ours, it is the Lords.

I know you have probably heard Yolanda Adams sing, "The Battle Is Not Yours" or you have heard that saying before, but you have yet to put it into practice. Well, let us discuss how to finally get victory in your battles.

The wise king Solomon wrote in Proverbs 3:5-6, *"Trust in the LORD with all thine heart; and lean not unto thine own understanding. In all thy ways acknowledge him, and he shall direct thy paths."*[27]

---

25   King James Version
26   King James Version
27   King James Version

The difficulty is that many women have been hurt repeatedly, and have yet to heal from these hurts and pains. Many women believe that their healing has to take a backseat to coping. You made the decision that life must go on and that you just could not put your life, your marriage, your children, your job, your ministry on hold to heal from your pain. This, however, was your decision and not God's. Allowing God to direct your paths means you have to let Him drive and you must move over into the passenger seat. Due to the rejection and betrayal of people in your past, you attempt to ensure your happiness by driving yourself there. The problem is, however, you will never get there by yourself. You cannot arrive at happiness or joy unless God brings you there. God will not take you there until He purges you of the tendencies that you can't use at the next level of your journey.

In the metamorphosis of a monarch butterfly, the caterpillar goes through a process of shedding feet and skin that will hinder its aviation. Similarly, GOD needs to subject you to a process of healing where he purges you of the bitterness, the fear, and desire for self-glory. He knows those attributes hinder your destiny. The battle is the Lord's; however, GOD commissions us to be soldiers in His army and to do some fighting as well. Your fight is three-fold.

1) Fight the urge to faint.

Giving up, especially in the midst of a terrible storm is tempting. However, you must hold on to the promise that trouble will not last always, and joy comes in the morning. Mastering endurance is the best preparation for success. In the movie *Coach Carter* starring Samuel L. Jackson, Carter took over as the basketball coach of a local high school. The team was eager to learn offensive plays and even defensive plays; however, the first thing that he taught them was endurance. He made the team run and run and run until he developed their endurance. Endurance is a function of the will. You have to make up your mind that you won't give up. Many people ask me what is the secret to the success of my marriage. Next to the grace of God working in our marriage, I attribute the success to our endurance. For me, divorce is not an option. Before we even got engaged, we agreed that divorce was something that was unacceptable to us. Consequently, we made up our minds **before** we got married, that we would endure the trials and tribulations of marriage until death do us part. So before you begin whatever journey you are embarking on, make up in your mind that fainting is not an option.

2) Fight the reliance on your own strength.

The Apostle Paul says that GOD's strength is made perfect in our weakness.[28] It suggests that GOD is actually attracted to our weakness and repelled by our strength. We marvel about how strong and independent many African American women are; however, it is imperative that you rely less on your own strength and more on the power of GOD. You must readily and sincerely admit, "I am weak." This truth is very difficult to internalize for women who pride themselves on being very strong and independent. However, the key to tapping into the power of God is in the relationship and partnership we have with Him. Having a low estimation of yourself is better than esteeming yourself too highly. If you are full of pride, or have a feeling of self-sufficiency, then you won't ask for help. Consequently, you will fight your own battles until you faint. The apostle James says in James 4:6 that "*GOD gives more grace.*"[29] If you humble yourself, GOD will give you the grace (unmerited favor) to be successful. The reality is that like Joseph you are in a pit. Either you have placed yourself into a pit, or someone else has placed you into a pit. You do not have the strength or the wherewithal to get yourself out. You need help. It is imperative that you learn how to relinquish control and wait for God to deliver you out of that pit at his appointed time. Listen to the emotional testimony of David: "*I love the Lord, because He has heard my voice and my supplications. Because He has inclined His ear to me, therefore I will call upon Him as long as I live. The pains of*

28   II Corinthians 12:9 (King James Version)
29   New King James Version

death surrounded me, and the pangs of Sheol laid hold of me; I found trouble and sorrow. Then I called upon the name of the Lord: 'O Lord, I implore You, deliver my soul!' Gracious is the Lord, and righteous; Yes, our God is merciful. The Lord preserves the simple; I was brought low and he saved me."[30] David's testimony is that he, like you, was brought low and God delivered him out of his low place. Implicit in that statement was that David couldn't deliver himself, but had to rely on the grace and strength of GOD.

3) Fight temptation.

I would contend that most people believe that we are either tempted by GOD or tempted by the devil. We are not tempted by God, and while we are often tempted by the devil, more often than not, we are also tempted by our own lusts. It is true that we are tested by GOD, but not with the purpose of sinning. GOD's purpose for testing us is to develop our patience which is a step in our maturation process. A temptation is something altogether different. A temptation is not a temptation unless it is attainable and desirable. In other words, if we want something and it is attainable, then we can be tempted by that thing. If I was fasting and you tried to tempt me with some chitterlings, I would not be tempted because I don't like nor eat chitterlings. However, if you put some fried chicken in front of me, then I am an easy target. All the devil does is to present opportunities for us to act on our own lusts. If we didn't lust after the desires of our own flesh, then the devil would not be such a successful co-conspirator. You need to understand that lust is a function of our flesh or our carnal nature. We are born into this world with the predisposition to satisfy the desires of our flesh. Therefore, the devil has carte blanche to present opportunities for us to act on our desires. However, since we are weak we often get in trouble. Even after we receive salvation, we still have our sinful nature, but now we also have a Holy nature. We now have two natures warring with one another. Paul in his letter to the

---

30   Psalms 116:1-6 (New King James Version)

Galatian church says that *"if we sow to the flesh we will reap corruption; but, if we sow to the Spirit we will reap everlasting life."*[31] The enemy (tempter) wants to lead us down a path that leads to a corrupt life. A life full of pain, anxiety, and misery is an example of a corrupt life. It is corrupt because it robs you of life's true vitality: which is love, peace, and joy. Consequently, that is what forgiveness offers. It offers love, peace, and joy.

Now, forgiveness is not something our flesh desires. It is contrary to human nature. Naturally speaking, if you hurt me, I desire to hurt you back. If you talk about me, I desire to talk about you. Hence, for you to really forgive, it means that you must fight the temptation to respond to the offense out of your flesh's desires. Instead, you must allow your inner-man to be led by the Holy Spirit to heal and to forgive. This point is very significant. How many times have women, who have been cheated on by their husbands, commited adultery out of revenge? How many times have you allowed your tongue (words) to reciprocate for the hurt you have received? One of the more prevalent themes in the Bible is forgiveness. Unfortunately, many women are ready to fight because of the intense pain that they feel. Hence, they seek out whom they can destroy. First, their motivation is wrong.

Any time you are motivated by vengeance, it is always the wrong motive. Second, this strategy is not effective. When you employ this strategy, it is you who will be destroyed. You must be led by Jehovah Rohi (The Lord my shepherd) to the destination that God has intended for you. On the one hand it seems therapeutic to get even or to get back at the offender. But, the reality is that your flesh is not *satisfied*, only *gratified*.

As mentioned earlier, there is a difference between being satisfied and being gratified. I am convinced that a real understanding between the two would prevent a great deal of adultery and other problems in marriages. For many people, anger, bitterness, and revenge seem pleasurable even if only for a moment.

Revenge provides temporary gratification, but forgiveness

---

31   Galatians 6:8 (New King James Version)

provides eternal satisfaction. The fight is to starve your flesh and feed your spirit. Practically speaking, this means avoid hanging out with your friends who are going to tell you to act on your lustful desires. It means putting someone in place who will hold you accountable. It means changing your email address or cell phone number if that is what it takes. It specifically means seeking the will of GOD and understanding your proper response based on the fruit of the Spirit. The truth of the matter is that the same power that raised Jesus from the dead is the same power that is available to every Christian. The problem, however, is that we use this resurrection power to raise the power of sin in our lives. When Jesus gave up the ghost, he destroyed the power of sin. So what do we do, we bring it back. Why? We bring it back because we are more comfortable controlling the old than allowing ourselves to be controlled by the new. The reality is that we never controlled the old, but rather we were controlled by our old nature. It may seem like you had control, but it was only an illusion of control. The old way of fighting has proven repeatedly not to work. You must begin a different fight!

One of the greatest fights recorded in the Bible in my opinion is recorded in I Samuel 30 when David and his men return to Ziklag only to find it besieged and ransacked. I posit that this is one of the greatest fights recorded in history because David was undoubtedly tempted in the aforementioned three areas. I am sure he was tempted to faint. I am sure he wanted to take matters in his own hands. And I am sure he wanted to exact revenge on all the people who hated on him, doubted him, and stole from him. Finally, I am sure David was tempted to act on his lustful desires and to be prideful.

When David and his men returned to Ziklag, they realized that they had not just lost their material possessions, but their most prized possessions, their wives and children. As Kirk Franklin would say, this was the fight of David's life. It is one thing to fight to rescue and restore Israel's reputation from the Philistines by defeating Goliath; however, it is another thing when you have lost your dignity, the respect of other people, and most importantly, your family. David did four things that assured him the victory in his fight. I am persuaded that if you employ these principles in your fight, you can also receive the victory.

1) Purpose to emote.

When David and his men came back to Ziklag to find everything gone, the first thing they did was weep until they had no more power to weep. Mary J. Blige is a successful R&B singer; and it is well noted that her depression and fight with low self esteem, addiction, and unforgiveness caused her to shed many tears. She got to a place in her career where she started recording songs like, "Not Gon Cry" and "No More Drama." And many women such as you, the one reading this book, have probably shed a great deal of tears in your lifetime. Consequently, you may have arrived to the point where you just do not want to cry any more. You may feel that weeping is useless and only brings you down. You may be emotionally constipated, and need help in letting the tears flow. In other words, you must prioritize and pursue emoting as an essential strategy to winning the fight. Emoting does two major things. First, it opens up your heart. Opening up your heart brings you to the place of weakness. As explained earlier, GOD is attracted to weakness; hence, this is essential in our attempt to connect with GOD. Second, emoting allows the expression of pain. Too often, many women drink, smoke, have sex, resent, or eat their pain away. These are unhealthy coping mechanisms. Emoting is a healthy and effective way to express hurts and pains. You may be thinking that David had no time to weep because his family had been taken captive. David understood that weeping was the first order of business. Now, it is possible to grieve inordinately. When excessive grieving leads to lack of motivation, then it is not beneficial, but rather destructive. Healthy emoting will always lead to positive action.

2) Pray for encouragement.

The Bible states that David *"encouraged himself in the Lord His God."*[32] The Hebrew word translated "encouraged" literally means to *fasten*. In other words, David fastened himself or attached himself to God in order to receive encouragement. When you read that scripture, it almost seems that David did all of the work and gave himself a pep talk because it says that David encouraged himself. The key is in the last five words of verse 6. The last five words are *"in the Lord his God."* [33] This lets us know that David received encouragement in the context of his personal relationship with his God. One of the best ways to receive encouragement or strengthening is by prayer. In Psalm 27, David says *"wait on the Lord and be of good courage and He shall strengthen your heart."* Isaiah 40 says *"wait on the Lord and He will renew your strength."* The Hebrew word for *wait* in both of these scriptures is *kaava*. It also literally means to bind together or to fasten. So after you weep and emote, then you must pray for encouragement. Specifically, pray for the strength and courage to fight and to endure. Paul says in Ephesians 6:10 *"Be strong in the Lord and in the power of His might."* [34] Take advantage of the awesome power of GOD by communing with Him.

3) Seek perfect enlightenment.

I initially thought that after David received encouragement from GOD, he would be ready to go after his enemies. However, David did something that seemed strange. He went to Abiather the priest and requested the ephod. The ephod was a priestly garment that had attached to it what was called the breastplate of judgment. Inside the breastplate of judgment was the Urim and Thummim, meaning "lights" and "perfections" respectively. In Old Testament times, sometimes GOD would give revelation concerning judgment by the Urim and

---

32   I Samuel 30:6 (King James Version)
33   I Samuel 30:6(King James Version)
34   King James Version

Thummim. Some Biblical scholars believe the Urim and Thummim to be a type of oracle. David understood that it was not enough to weep, and it was not enough to have encouragement. He understood that you also need enlightenment. Many women have strength to fight; however, because they don't have GOD's perfect enlightenment they go in the wrong direction with the wrong motivation. The Bible is God's perfect enlightenment and should be consulted before engaging in battle. The Bible is a lamp unto your feet and a light unto your path. A lamp lets you know where you are, but a light illuminates the path to where you are going. Your steps need be ordered by the Lord. In addition, God has anointed certain people to be wise and endowed with the gift of counsel. They help you understand the Bible and help to guide you in the right direction. These persons can illuminate not just your problems, but also the path to your solution.

There are two main paths, the path that God has ordained for us and the path that we ordain for ourselves. Typically, on the path we choose, there are very few obstacles visible to the naked eye. Logically speaking, that path seems like the best route to take. The path God would have you to take, however, has many obstacles visible to the naked eye, but it also has the angels of God (invisible to the naked eye) all around. The only way you would walk down this road is if you walked by faith. John 16:3 says that *"the Spirit will guide us into all truth."*[35] This is a major point because there is a way that seems right; however, the ends are the ways of death. What do I mean practically by death? I mean the death of healthy relationships, the abortion of unborn potential, and decline in physical and spiritual health. Therefore, after you receive encouragement, it is vital that you receive enlightenment by the Holy Spirit and the Bible. God will lead you to people that can help you. In this story about Ziklag, God leads David to a man that takes them to the enemy's camp. When you allow God to direct your paths, He will lead you to someone that can help you. There is still one more thing you have to do to become victorious.

---

35   King James Version

4) Pursue the enemy.

For those who think that the process of forgiveness is passive, you are sorely mistaken. Forgiveness is an active fight that necessitates pursuing the enemy. I have many clients who, for years, passively waited for their oppressors and victimizers to apologize to them for the wounds that they inflicted on them. Some of those perpetrators are sleeping well at night not bothered by their offenses. Others are too sick, deranged, or too prideful to apologize. But while you are waiting, you are growing increasingly bitter. Not just towards them, but you are bitter, angry and cynical about life. Instead of this bitterness, you must target that which is slowly killing you. If you knew you had a tumor in your body, you would go after that tumor to destroy it with all haste and with all power at your disposal. Likewise, unforgiveness is a tumor that slowly kills many people. Hence, when you forgive, you are pursuing your internal enemy. Well, who is the enemy? When you think of enemy, what immediately come to many women's minds are their ex-husbands, their abusers, their bosses, parents, and the people who have betrayed their trust.

One of the major enemies that you need to pursue is unforgiveness. Just as David pursued the culprit that stole his family and possessions from him, you must target unforgiveness—the culprit which as taken your peace, your joy, your sleep, your health and your livelihood away from you. The story states that David and his 600 men pursued the enemy. When they came to the Brook Besor, 200 of the men fainted. David and the other 400 kept going. The men were led to their enemies. They fought until they recovered everything. On the way back from the battle, some of David's men said to him that the 200 who fainted and deserted them in battle should not partake in the blessing of the victory. But David rejected that notion and decided to bless even the deserters. He did this because he had the ability to forgive the people who had let him down.

Just as David purposed to emote, prayed for encouragement, sought perfect enlightenment, and pursued the enemy, which resulted in David recovering everything he had lost, it is now time for you to win the fight of your life. Are you ready for this fight? Are you ready to take back everything that was taken from you? You may be thinking I can't regain everything that was taken from me. I can't take my virginity, my innocence, and my childhood back. They were taken from me and they are gone. Like David, you might be tempted to seek revenge as you lament what was taken from you. Through his traumatic struggle, however, David overcame his temptations and was victorious. He was victorious because he was able to forgive. Furthermore, just as God gave Job double for his trouble, He will do the same for you. You must fight a different fight, though. It is important to note that Job received double only after he forgave the very people who attacked his character.[36]

---

36   Job 42:10 (King James Version)

Are you at the point in your life where you are tired of fighting? Look back over your life and list in detail the heavyweight fights you fought in your own strength. Describe the victories and the defeats.

_____

_____

_____

_____

_____

_____

_____

_____

_____

_____

_____

_____

_____

_____

_____

_____

_____

_____

_____

_____

_____

_____

To Trust or Not to Trust

"Soon as I stopped worrying, worrying how it was going to end."[37]

Trust in the Lord with all thy heart and lean not on your own understanding.[38]

IT IS UNDERSTANDABLE why Melissa chose to be a lesbian. It makes sense because most of the men in her life left a terrible impression on her. First, her father abandoned her when he found out that his girlfriend was pregnant. Then, Melissa was molested at age five by her uncle on several occasions, and was violently raped when she was fifteen. That was just the beginning. She thought she had fallen in love with a man at age 19 because of the attention and seeming comfort that he gave her; it felt like love. She did anything to keep this so-called love. She was extremely beautiful, and her greatest physical asset was her smile.

How could she project a smile in the midst of so much pain and turmoil? Well, after her boyfriend used her to fulfill his sexual needs, he then used her to fulfill his financial needs, along with his need for dominance and control. He demanded that she sell her body for money. She wanted to please him and she was desperate to keep him. She

---

37   Encourage Yourself (Donald Lawrence)
38   Proverbs 3:5 (King James Version)

did not know if she could live without him. This went on for years. No Good Samaritan saw her wounds. No pastor, no missionary; no one came to her rescue. Melissa even wondered why GOD didn't come to her rescue. One day, a woman saw her and was attracted to her. The woman was not necessarily attracted to Melissa's physical beauty, but rather she was attracted to her pain. She befriended Melissa and began to nurture her as a mother nurtures a child. They became partners and, for the first time in her life, Melissa thought she had joy. What Melissa realized however, was that her girlfriend had many issues herself. She was just as controlling as her ex-boyfriend/pimp. She realized that even though she had changed genders, she had attracted the same type of person. She had attracted the type of person who wanted to use her for their own selfish gain. Melissa became increasingly suicidal and desperately wanted an end to the misery. She went back to prostitution in order to survive. Fortunately, she was arrested. The judge gave her probation and ordered mandatory therapy. Her therapist happened to be a male. Initially, she resisted because of her intense negative feelings towards men. However, this psychotherapist cared for her and had her best interest at heart. He was not attracted to her and did not want anything from her. Instead, he wanted her to tap into her dormant intuitive ability to trust the healing process. He told her, "I know you do not trust anybody. You really do not even trust yourself, but in time you will realize that you have the ability to trust." What Melissa did not understand at the time was the correlation between a controlling spirit and the inability to trust.

Many women have been labeled "controlling." Either you fit the description, or you know someone who fits this description. While there are times when it is beneficial to act in control of a situation, it is unhealthy for control to become your permanent disposition. Whether intentionally or unintentionally, when you do not have regular bowel movements, you will become constipated. While the immediate effects of constipation are uncomfortable and painful, the long term effects of constipation are deadly. Medically speaking, when you are constipated, the accumulated waste in your colon forms a hard, solid mass. Only the waste that gets around this solid mass will be able to be moved out of the colon. The most effective treatment to combat this problem is to soften or break up the hard mass so the waste can be pushed out of your colon.

Likewise, many women are emotionally and spiritually constipated. They are emotionally constipated because they have let unresolved hurts and pains harden in their hearts. Consequently, they are unable to release these feelings without assistance. The years of unresolved hurts and pains have grown and formed a solid emotional mass which requires help in breaking it down. Although many women eventually come to grips with the fact that they have "unresolved issues," the problem is actually relinquishing control, which involves trust.

One of the greatest tragedies that befall many women is the loss of trust. Due to being abandoned, misused, and abused, the natural instinct to trust is often substituted with a need to control. Now, on the one hand, it is healthy to want to stop the drama and take matters into your own hands. It makes logical sense that if you keep on getting hurt in relationships, then you should pull back and isolate yourself to prevent more pain. While that step is necessary for growth, it is not the final nor is it the most important step. In the illustration of constipation, controlling your diet is extremely important in lessening its constipation's deleterious effects. Even though the diet is very important, the most efficacious treatment is to get rid of the waste that is already there. However, many people who are constipated do not like to make regular bowel movements. Some reasons for this include being time-consuming, uncomfortable and sometimes very painful. Avoiding having bowel movements on a regular basis is a demonstration of controlling the situation to avoid pain. Emotionally speaking, many women attempt to control their pain by refusing to deal with years of unresolved hurts. This avoidance makes it virtually impossible to trust.

Underneath the baggage, behind the control, and on top of the drama is not the *inability* to trust, but rather a conscious decision not to trust. The truth is that everyone has the ability to trust. The question becomes in whom or in what are you placing your trust. For many women, the

object of their trust is themselves. I know that you say you trust GOD and trust some people, but this trust to which you refer is the type of trust that is expressed when God and people agree with you. However, when GOD tells you to do something that is uncomfortable (like let go of your burdens, or let go of ungodly relationships), or that makes no logical sense, do you still trust GOD or do you trust you?

A baby comes into this world already wired to trust. Being able to trust is an innate characteristic that every human being is born with. That is one of the main reasons why a baby cries. She believes or "trusts" that someone will hear her cry and respond to her needs. Well, how and when does the breakdown of innate trust occur? The breakdown occurs when the people in whom we trust betray our confidence in them. One of the most damaging betrayals of trust is when a mother does not love and bond effectively with her child. In my practice, I see the results of this phenomenon frequently. I see many adult women having major difficulties in many (if not all) of their relationships; and, even as adults they do not trust that their mother really loves them or has ever had their best interest at heart.

Similarly, another major betrayal of trust is when "Daddy" betrays his daughter's trust. What an awesome opportunity to shape the worldview of his daughter by loving her, affirming her, protecting her, and modeling a healthy relationship by loving and being faithful to her mother. Unfortunately, with the epidemic of fatherlessness, abuse, and adultery, the trust that girls should have in men is shattered with every unhealthy relationship that they see and experience. Hence, many girls grow up witnessing the intense pain of their mothers at the hand of the fathers (or other men) and subsequently develop less and less trust for men.

So, to trust or not to trust, that is the question. Well, we have already explained that everybody has the innate ability to trust. The question is *whom* should you trust? Spiritually speaking, Psalms 118:8

says, *"It's better to trust in the Lord than to put confidence in man."*[39] When the Bible speaks of man in this verse, it is not only referring to males. Since we all trust in something or somebody, it is better to trust in GOD than in people or princes. However, GOD still wants you to trust certain people to an extent. Proverbs 24:6 declares that *"there is safety in the multitude of wise counselors."*[40] In other words, there are some wise people who are worthy of your trust. Another example of this is found in James 5:16, where James teaches us that we must *"confess our faults one to another."*[41] The implication in this verse is that you are confessing your faults to someone trustworthy, and not someone who does not have the skill or discretion to keep your personal matters private. There are some individuals with whom you should share nothing personal at all. These people are easy to spot, for they are the ones that are always gossiping and minding everyone else's business except for their own. Remember Joseph the dreamer told his brothers his dream and they put him in a pit.

Restoring Trust

The key to restoring the ability to trust is two fold: 1) knowing who to trust and 2) knowing how to trust. The following paragraphs will provide practical guidance on who to trust and how to trust.

Who to Trust

You are probably in a relationship wondering whether you should trust this potential boyfriend, fiancé, or husband. There are so many people who have mastered the art of deception, such that many women find themselves repeating the same drama over and over again.

Godly people — Godly people are defined as people in whom the Spirit of GOD is visible and evident by spiritual fruit. Notice that I did

---

39   King James Version
40   King James Version
41   King James Version

not say that Godly people are the ones who say that they are Godly. That is a red flag. Be leery if someone says, "You can trust me," or "I am spiritual." Godly people don't have to convince people that they are Godly--the proof is in the pudding. The proof is in their demonstration of godliness. These people express the fruit of the spirit: love, peace, joy, meekness, gentleness, goodness, temperance, longsuffering, and patience. If you let the Holy Spirit order your steps, you will be led to these types of people. There is an expression that says, "The dog that brings the bone carries the bone." It means, when observing someone's fruit, if they have ever brought gossip (the bone) to you, they are likely to disclose your confidential information to others. The Holy Spirit in you will recognize the Holy Spirit in Godly people.

Dependable people — When you find yourself in a crisis, you will need to trust someone for help. One sure fire way to know if someone is dependable is to depend on them. If the stakes are too high in a particular situation, then you need to first look at that person's track record. If he/she has been consistently dependable, then she/he may be worthy of your trust. It is wise to be led to people who have proven to be dependable over a variety of different situations and circumstances. As a father of five children, I have become a connoisseur of diapers. You name it I have purchased them from Huggies to Pampers, to Luvs to various supermarket brands. Sometimes I would purchase a certain brand solely based on price. However, when my child woke my wife and me up at 3am because his diaper had leaked, I decided I was willing to pay more for dependable diapers. Similarly, dependable people will prove to be valuable and will separate themselves from the rest, even if it costs you more time in searching them out.

Wise people — Wisdom is the opposite of folly. Folly is the behavior of fools. Don't look for people who have the potential to be wise. Rather, look for the abundance of wisdom already evident in their lives. One of the definitions of wisdom in the Hebrew tongue is skillful. I often tell people not to tell everyone or just anyone your problems, because most people don't know what to do or how to handle your issues let alone their own. One of the best pieces of evidence of a skillful person I their ability to keep matters private. Solomon in Proverbs 25:2 says that *"it is the glory of God to conceal a matter."*[42] A wise person not only has wisdom in terms of guidance and direction, but they can keep information confidential. Keeping information confidential is a skill not everyone possesses. I have seen people promise with sincerity that they would keep information private. By the end of the day, they had told the private information. Some people just have to tell it. They just can't help themselves. A wise person will also have good information to share and they are practicing what they are preaching. I would not seek marital advice from some someone who has been divorced four times. He/she obviously does not know how to have a successful marriage. The Bible says that wisdom is justified of her children. In other words, a person who is wise produces wise fruit.

How to Trust

Now that we know *who* to trust, I will discuss *how* to trust. Webster's definition of trust is "assured reliance on the character, ability, strength, or truth of someone or something."[43] Now this seems pretty simple doesn't it? Well, it would be simple if the people whom you are supposed to trust demonstrated these characteristics clearly. Trusting nowadays for many women often is like rolling the dice. There actually is wisdom regarding how to trust that is rarely practiced in relationships. Yet, if more women employ the following principles, their lives would be filled with joy. The following section provides practical steps on how to trust.

1) **Reveal** the source of the problem. The word *reveal* is derived from the Latin word, "revelare," which means to uncover. This is significant because the real problems in relationships are not evident, but instead are latent or hidden. When a husband cheats on his wife, the problem is not that he is unfaithful. The infidelity is merely a symptom

---

42   King James Version
43   Webster's Collegiate Dictionary

of the problem. One of the major problems in relationships is that we spend too much time focusing on the symptoms and not on the actual source of the problem. In psychology we call this phenomenon "symptom substitution." If you spend the majority of your time eradicating the symptom, then a new symptom will emerge to replace the symptom that was eradicated. However, the source of the problem has yet to be dealt with. As an illustration, after the woman finds out or suspects that her husband has cheated on her, she gets angry at him. Soon after the anger subsides, she begins to blame herself. She asks herself, "What did I do wrong?" Am I good enough or pretty enough?" If you have ever asked yourself that question, know that you are not the problem. Well, you are not *his* problem. His problem(s) occurred before the relationship.

The primary mistake made in this scenario is that the woman ignored the symptom. Understanding the symptoms leads to what and where the source of the problem is. For example, if you have frequent chest pains, it behooves you to investigate whether these symptoms point to an underlying problem. If these pains are ignored, death becomes very possible. Likewise, in the example of infidelity, when you first know that your significant other is unfaithful, don't assume that the symptom is the problem, but rather investigate it immediately to uncover the problem. Trained cardiologists conduct a series of tests to discover that there is a blocked artery. Likewise, you must employ a series of invasive and intrusive tests to root out the source of the problem. Several factors may contribute to that problem; some, however, are out of your control. For example, in the case of his infidelity, one major source of the problem may be that he does not trust you enough to meet his needs. That is *his* issue. He, in fact, has a trust problem. Do not spend countless hours focusing on insignificant information like who she was and what she looks like. Recognize that he has a major trust issue that, if not resolved, will kill the relationship. You may say well he has more issues than trust. Well, if he does not trust you or God enough to confess and to ask for help, then it still boils down to trust. It is important to understand that this problem has to be uncovered. It is not easily seen. Your significant other will probably not say, "The problem is that I have major trust issues and I don't know if I can trust you to meet my needs." With illumination from the Holy Spirit and wise counsel, you will uncover this problem. After you reveal the problem, you then have two choices.

2) Run or Restore. When the problem is revealed, you can either *run* from the relationship or *restore* the relationship. It is disappointing to see that the women who are supposed to run actually stay; and, the women who are supposed to restore their relationships actually run. If you are not married to him, then run. I hear you saying, "But what if I love him?" My response would be, "Then love him from a distance." You cannot fix his trust problem. If you believe that GOD has ordained you to be together, then tell him that you will wait for him to heal so you can be together. If a man is serious, he will seek help, and then come after you. Many women, unfortunately, because of their own trust issues do not demand and expect spiritual maturity from their mates. Many women don't trust GOD to send them someone who will be faithful and trustworthy.

So instead of GOD picking your mate, you pick your mate. I learned a long time ago, however, that I was not wise enough to pick my own mate. I did not know her past and I did not know her future, but God does. Since GOD does not make mistakes, when I chose the one He chose for me, I knew I couldn't go wrong.

On the other hand, if you are married, then running should not be your first option. You should seek wise counsel immediately to help uncover the depth of the problem so that you can apply immediate pressure to resolving it. The solution to this problem is called *restoration*. Restoration is a process where those who are disjointed become unified. Marriage is supposed to be a process where two individuals become one entity. Let's look at the mathematics of marriage. One times one equals one. Marriage is not about addition, but rather multiplication. The difficulty, however, is that the aforementioned equation presupposes that both the groom and the bride are whole persons at the time of marriage. The reality, however, is that most marriages involve two half-way whole people coming together. Now let's do the math. One half times one half is actually one fourth. This is profound! In other words, when two incomplete people join in marriage, you start off the marriage worse off then when you were single. When you were single, at least you were half-way whole. Now both of you combined are a quarter whole. Hence, restoration involves addressing the baggage that you bring into the marriage. In other words, you must become *whole* individually before your marriage can be restored.

The priority of the restoration is first vertical before horizontal. Your relationship with God must be restored before your marriage can be restored. The vertical relationship empowers the horizontal relationship. This is very important because many wives are looking to their husbands to show them tangible proof of change before they will begin their own restorative process. The reality is that both spouses probably won't actively work on restoring their relationship with God at the same time. So, if you are waiting on your spouse to change before you change, you are missing the point. Here is the overarching principle: once you learn how to really trust and depend on God, He will direct you to stay or go. If God directs you to stay, He will provide enough grace, wisdom, and endurance to be at peace even while your spouse has yet to change.

Identify the people you can trust according to criteria described in this chapter.

_____

_____

_____

_____

_____

_____

_____

_____

_____

_____

_____

_____

_____

_____

_____

_____

_____

_____

_____

_____

_____

_____

Fears for Tears

A cry is a sorrowful thing; it is the language of pain. (Charles Spurgeon)

Shout, shout let it all out; these are the things I can do without.[44]

CAMILLE WAS THE type of woman who wore her emotions on her sleeve. She could not hide her true feelings even if she wanted to. It just so happened that the predominant emotion that Camille expressed was anger. She was always agitated, frequently frustrated, and usually unkind; but, this was the perception of the casual observer. She had earned a reputation for being mean, cold, callous, uncaring, dude-like, and the list went on and on. Unfortunately, most of the people who encountered Camille, did not see underneath the exterior, but instead looked at the cover and judged her. Underneath the stone-cold exterior, however, was a fragile and delicate heart. Camille was not as confident or as tough as her exterior communicated; instead, she was unsure of her value and deeply fearful. She was fearful about whether she would ever be successful, she was fearful about life in general, and fearful about whether she would ever be happy.

She was tough, not because she wanted to be, but because she

---

44   "Shout" (Tears For Fears)

felt she had to be. From a young age her mother modeled self-reliance, toughness, and inculcated that it was foolish and moronic to depend on a man. Camille's mother felt justified in teaching her daughter this principle because Camille's father abandoned his marriage and his children, and all of the family responsibilities had fallen on her. Publically, Camille's mother never shed a tear and she vowed that everything would be alright. Camille's mother repeatedly told her, "Crying is useless; it does not solve anything. Crying is for weak people." Despite this instruction, Camille was a crier. She just could not help herself. Camille was extremely sensitive and emotional. The least bit of disapproval and anger from her mother provoked Camille to tears. This angered Camille's mother immensely.

When Camille turned 14 years old, she made up her mind that she would have to change to gain her mother's approval. She decided that if she were cold, callous, and in control of her emotions, her mother would accept her and be proud of her. Unfortunately, Camille's plan did not work. Camille became just like her mother; angry, bitter, lonely, and unfulfilled. Camille also became extremely anxious, fearful, and unable to trust anyone. After the breakup of her last relationship, Camille began to face her issues, and she decided to seek help.

During our counseling session, Camille began to talk about her childhood; and choked up. However, she willed herself not to cry. I could see the frustration on her face as the tears began to form in her eyes. Of course, I encouraged her to cry for that was part of the healing process. With an angry tone she responded, "I don't want to cry!" This refusal to cry lasted for five sessions, for she had willed herself to talk cognitively and intellectually about deeply painful things, but not to emote. No matter how many times I explained to her that part of the healing process entails expressing the deep hurts by crying, Camille did not budge. Yet, her eventual healing was inextricably tied to her ability to relent and let it out.

There was a popular rock/pop song in the 1980's called "Shout," performed by a group called "Tears for Fears." The chorus of the song says, *"Shout, shout, let it all out; these are things I can do without;*

Come on, I'm talking to you; Come on". The theme of that song should be an unspoken anthem for healing. Simply put, there needs to be a profound exchange or transfer by women of their fears for tears. Now this exchange may not make sense because transfers or exchanges usually involve two or more people. But, in the healing process that is exactly what takes place. Jesus said, *"Take my yoke upon you and learn from Me, for I am gentle and lonely in heart, and you will find rest for your souls. My yoke is easy and My burden is light."*[45] Jesus is explaining the divine transfer for healing. Jesus is encouraging you to give Him your fears, anxieties, stress, and burdens and he will give you rest. Also 1 Peter 5:7 says, *"Casting all your care upon him; for he cares for you."*[46] Rest is synonymous with healing. Many physicians encourage their recovering patients to rest, to permit the medicine and the body's natural immune forces to restore the body. In fact, the restoration and rebuilding process only occurs during rest periods. Similarly, when you exchange your fears with the Lord and take His burden, you specifically give permission for the Holy Spirit to purge, purify, and restore you. Here is the point: this healing process will produce involuntary crying.

The common response to crying is that it makes people feel weak. Bingo! God's strength is made perfect in our weakness. Weakness is good in the right context. Three processes occur during this exchange: 1) catharsis; 2) comforting; and 3) conquering.

1) Catharsis is a word derived from the Greek word *katharsis* which means purging or cleansing. Purging or cleansing involves extracting or removing something out. As it relates to crying, catharsis involves the expressing or the extracting of pain out of the system. When a mother extracts milk out of her breast when engorged, she experiences tremendous relief. Many women are engorged, but not with milk, with guilt, pain, and shame. When these hurts are expressed out of the system, a catharsis will ensue.

---

45   Matthew 11:29,30 (New King James Version)
46   New King James Version

2) Comforting describes the second process that occurs during the aforementioned exchange. As the pain is being expressed, you are in the midst of the pain. You are not avoiding the pain, but rather you are purposefully engaging the pain in order to express or extract it out. This leaves the soul ripe for comfort. David in Psalm 34:18 reminds us that *"The LORD is near to those who have a broken heart, and saves such as have a contrite spirit."* Specifically, when one humbles herself, surrenders to the process of healing, and exchanges her burdens for the LORD's peace, the Holy Spirit or Comforter begins the purifying and extracting process. Now, while the extraction is painful, the presence of GOD and His consolation comforts you even during the painful process. It is one thing to go through this painful process alone, but GOD promises never to leave you nor forsake you. *Comforter* in the New Testament is translated from the Greek word "Paraclete and etymologically signifies "called to one's side." Since every Christian has the Comforter dwelling within, the potential for this support and comfort is always available. However, the strength or power of the Comforter is at its greatest in our weakness. I recommend the following prayer of support:

> *Dear Lord, I have come to the realization that I am weak and desperate. I have depended on myself for too long, and I am still broken. Please remove me out of the way, and allow Your Holy Spirit to heal me. Father, as you purge me of all of my pains and fears, be a balm for my wounds, and comfort me with your presence! In Jesus' name, Amen.*

3) Conquering is the third result of exchanging your burdens for the LORD's peace. Until this exchange however, fear rules the soul. The main reasons that many women merely cope rather than heal are the fear of how painful the process will be, and also the fear of losing control. Healing is an unpredictable process, and often times the pain is excruciating. The comfort of the healing process is that there is an end. If you can endure to the end, then the pain and the fear will no longer torment you.

Losing control involves lowering your defenses which will leave you vulnerable. You are indeed vulnerable to attack and disappointment; however, you are also vulnerable to the conquering power of GOD. Faith is the only thing that can overcome this deep-seated fear. One of the greatest weapons that Satan uses to defeat Christians is fear. The Bible says that GOD did not give us a spirit of fear. Well, if GOD did not give it to us, then where did it come from? It came from the enemy to torment us. 1 John 4:18 says, *there is no fear in love, but perfect love casts out all fear, because fear involves torment. But he who fears has not been made perfect in love.* Overcoming fear can only happen when you surrender to perfect love. When you say, "I am weak, but Thou art mighty" you (by faith) summon the power of GOD to act on your behalf. GOD in His perfect love begins to work in you and work for you to conquer any fear or issue in your life. That's why Romans 8:37 empowers us to know that we are more than conquerors through Him who *loved* us.

So let the tears flow. Initially, the tears will be tears of pain. However, when the Comforter starts the transformation process, He will transform the tears from tears of pain to tears of joy. He will turn your sorrow into joy and your mourning into dancing.

Describe why you don't like to cry. Who influenced your feelings regarding crying? What are your fears? Who influenced those fears? Are you ready to exchange your fears for tears?

_____

_____

_____

_____

_____

_____

_____

_____

_____

_____

_____

_____

_____

_____

_____

_____

_____

_____

_____

_____

_____

_____

_____

PART III
THE DELIVERANCE

The Gift that Keeps on Giving

To err is human, to forgive is divine

WHILE THIS PHRASE, "Let go and let GOD" is frequently repeated, it is rarely achieved. It makes perfect and logical sense to let the one with supreme power carry the burdens that are too heavy for our shoulders. I see the sincere desire to let go of these painful burdens, but it rarely happens. The culprit is a perceived need to "hold" and "control." Many Black women tend to hold to the issues in their lives and try to control them using their ingenuity and their efforts. The evidence is undeniable. Our realization of this phenomenon has grown to the point that Black women will now say, "I know I have control issues." Since awareness is the first step toward healing, let me validate the progress. Note that, at its core the tendency to control is a successful coping mechanism. Popular psychiatrist Freud would argue that the need to control is our way of preventing unwanted and unconscious impulses from becoming conscious. After being hurt, abused, and misused by many people, it seems healthy for a person to assume control of as many aspects of life as possible. This is why we have so many strong, independent Black women. I would dare to say that most Black women who are independent are so out of necessity rather than choice. This is because so many of them have been let down over and over again by people that, by definition, are supposed to be trustworthy, e.g. your mother, father, husband, and best friend.

The reality is that many women don't even trust themselves because they give and give and give, yet receive in return nothing but abuse, infidelity, lies, deceit, and pain. On one hand, it seems logical for Black women to take matters into their own hands. However, if the aforementioned patterns of abuse, infidelity, deceit, and pain continue, then "holding" and "controlling" are not effective. I tell strong, independent, African American clients of mine that being independent and controlling was actually necessary for an immediate change out of the dysfunction, but they have to learn how to trust again and how to depend on God and others again. The precursor to being able to trust again is forgiveness.

I call forgiveness the gift that keeps on giving. A popular jewelry store slogan is "Give the gift that keeps on giving," referring to diamonds. A popular quote is *diamonds last forever*. It is quite clever and effective marketing to suggest that women can have eternal happiness from the outside in. I would dare to say, however, that forgiveness is really the only gift that keeps on giving. Forgiveness is a spiritual gift and is antithetical to control. We are not born with the ability to truly forgive. To the contrary, it is our human nature to hold grudges and to demand payment for being wronged. Even if the only payment we require is justice, we still require something in return. On the other hand, forgiveness is a gift born of Agape love. As discussed in the foregoing section, it is an aspect of Godly love. Those who do not have Godly love living in them, really do not have the ability, desire, or wherewithal to forgive.

Popular psychology and the media paint an incorrect picture of what forgiveness looks like. They say, "Just forgive, forget, and move on." First of all, we really do not forget many things. God has created our brains to remember almost anything. Even when we experience trauma to our brains and suffer from amnesia, we can retrieve the memory under certain circumstances. This principle is analogous to trying to delete a file from the computer. Even after you decide to permanently delete a file, an IT specialist can retrieve what was thought to be permanently erased. Hence, we really do not forget the hurt and pain or the ones who inflicted this hurt and pain. But forgiveness allows the power or effect of the pain to be transformed into something good. Forgiveness also transforms the mind such that one looks at the experience differently. Have you ever been in a really nasty argument with your husband, broken up with your boyfriend, or been divorced? When you are in the midst of that pain, your thoughts regarding the relationship or man were almost all negative. Even after you cool down and the intensity of your pain diminishes, you still look at the relationship in a negative light. You may have taken the blame off of him, and placed it onto yourself. You say, "I can't believe I let him use me like that. How could I fall for that?" You may have transferred the negative feelings, but you are still bound by them. When you forgive, however, your view of the relationship will be more objective as you will be able to identify the positives and negatives of the relationship, and glean from them that you are better, stronger, and wiser because of the struggles.

Before we explore the true meaning of forgiveness, we first need to understand what it is not.

1) Forgiveness is not giving or receiving an apology.

When someone who has hurt you apologizes to you, even when it seems genuine, that does not constitute forgiveness. The process of forgiveness really does not involve apologizing to the other person. That process is called apologizing. While apologizing is very necessary, it is not forgiveness. Forgiveness is between you and God. Forgiveness can only happen when you have God's love living and operating in your life. Often times, God has to give us a greater measure of forgiveness in order to forgive those who have truly hurt us. I have worked with adult women who have been carrying burdens of guilt, unresolved anger, and other issues involving their parents. The burdens are so heavy that the clients genuinely desire to release them, but they erroneously believe that since their parents are deceased it is too late. It is not too late. As long as you are alive and alive in GOD, you have the capacity to truly forgive. Also, forgiveness empowers both you and the one that has harmed you. If you harbor pain and bitterness, you are not doing what Galatians 6:1 says: "*Brethren, if a man is overtaken in any trespass, you who spiritual restore such a one in a spirit of gentleness, considering yourself lest you also be tempted.*" [47] While forgiveness empowers both of you, it empowers the one who forgives in a greater way. Yes, relationally, the forgiven will be better off when you forgive him, but he might not have a clue that he needed to be forgiven. He might be living life with not a care in the world, sleeping peacefully, while you are up every night tossing and turning, feeling anxious and unsettled about what that person did. True forgiveness is when God takes the hurt and pain and transforms it into growth, maturity and power. That weight is removed and you are not only freed from the pain, but also freed from the shackles of those feelings.

2) Forgiveness is not failing to confront the one who hurt you.

Some people truly believe the misconception that "time heals all wounds." Time does not heal wounds, God does. And God will heal only if you allow Him to. Many women confront the one that hurt them by cursing them out, shattering their windshields, slashing their tires, cheating for revenge, etc. R&B singer Jasmine Sullivan has a song entitled, "Bust Your Windows" about a woman who reacts to being hurt by her man by busting the windows out of his car. Toward the end of the song she realizes that she is not really satisfied, nor over the pain.

Other women choose to try and not think about it, hoping that time will ease the pain. It is true, that these women may seem less angry and frustrated, but they have just internalized these emotions rather than expressed or externalized them. This is not forgiveness. Instead, it is the path to depression. Confronting pain is essential, but

---

47   New King James Verson

only during the process of forgiveness. Now, healthy confrontation is not violent or done from a vengeful spirit. It is the process of speaking with deep sincerity and honesty while targeting the source of the problem.

3) Forgiveness is not a psychological technique.

Discussions of forgiveness are becoming more popular in psychological literature. Even in *Jet*, *Essence*, and *Ebony* magazines, Black psychologists stated how forgiveness can positively impact one's emotional well-being. This information is accurate for the most part. The problem is that the whole story is not told, which leaves great room for error. Learning how to forgive is not something I read in a psychology textbook or something I learned in graduate school. While I am excited to see more researchers studying the scientific merits of forgiveness; the psychological literature only leads to the screen door of forgiveness. If you want to open the door of forgiveness, you need to keep knocking. True forgiveness must be understood in the context of its spiritual basis.

The Spiritual Basis of Forgiveness

Forgiveness is a spiritual gift, and to really understand forgiveness, one has to understand how it works spiritually. The following are three principles that help explain the spiritual basis and process of forgiveness.

1. Forgiveness begins with the Father

I read a popular magazine article recently about forgiveness. This article gave very tangible and concrete steps on how to forgive someone. On the surface it seemed like a wonderful and effective article. However, there was something noticeably absent from the article, which is the same thing that's absent when you turn on many talk shows that address forgiveness. The thing that is missing is the mentioning of God in the same context as the mentioning of forgiveness. In Luke 23:34, Jesus who is on the cross to be crucified, utters the first of the 7 Last Words, *"Father, forgive them; for they know not what they do."*[48] Notice that the first word that Jesus utters is not *forgive*, rather it is *Father*. Jesus demonstrates in Mark 2 that He has the power on earth to forgive sins. Why then would he ask his Father to forgive sins? Well, Jesus wanted to demonstrate and model how we ought to access the ability to forgive. The ability to forgive does not begin with us, it begins with God. James 1:17 states, *"every good and perfect gift comes from above, and comes down from the Father of lights, with whom there is no variation or shadow of turning."* [49] Forgiveness is a good and perfect gift. It is good because, by nature, forgiveness is beneficent and beneficial for all involved. It is perfect because it allows for the giver and the receiver of forgiveness to become perfect (mature). Therefore, the first thing you must do is ask the Father to help you to forgive.

2. Forgiveness is based on forgiveness

The second principle of forgiveness is that it is based on forgiveness. We do not have an innate ability, or capacity to forgive. Many Christians sing the song, "Oh, how I love Jesus, because he first loved me." Well those that have received this forgiveness can sing, "Oh, I can forgive, because he first forgave me." 1 Peter 4:10 says, *"As every man hath received the gift, even so minister the same one to another, as good stewards of the manifold grace of God."*[50] Therefore, because Christ forgave you, you have the ability and the authority to forgive others.

3. Forgiveness bears fruit

The third principle is that forgiveness bears fruit. Forgiveness is

---

48   New King James Version
49   New King James Version
50   King James Version

the miracle fruit. I am sure that you have heard of fruits such as Noni, Acai, Mangosteen, and Gogi-berry. There even is a product called Miracle Fruit Berry that temporarily rewires how your palate perceives sour flavors, rendering lemons sweet like candy.[51] There have been widespread claims that all these fruits can affect miraculous healing; however, forgiveness is a thousand times more miraculous.

When Jesus was on the cross, He was situated between two male-factors. When he said, *"Father forgive them,"*[52] who was he talking about? Was He referring to the malefactors on each side of Him? Was He referring to Pilate? Was He referring to the guards who were about to gamble for His garments, or was He referring to his disciples? To whom was He referring? I believe He was referring to all who were guilty. Those that are aware of their guilt and confess their sins, how-ever, can receive that forgiveness. 1 John 1:9 says, *"If we confess our sins, he is faithful and just to forgive us our sins, and to cleanse us from all unrighteousness."* [53] What is important to understand is that forgiveness is not just subtractive only. When Jesus forgave me, not only did He take my sins away and release me from debt and the penalty of my sins, but He also restored me. He gave me something valuable. He gave me His Spirit, and *"where the Spirit of the Lord is, there is liberty."*[54] Forgiveness is a fruit of the spirit, and Christians are the fruit that the forgiveness of Jesus produces. Must He bear the cross alone though? Jesus taught in the Lord's Prayer that God will forgive our debts as we forgive our debtors. He also said, *"For if ye forgive men their trespasses, your heavenly Father will also forgive you: But if ye forgive not men their trespasses, neither will your Father forgive your trespasses."*[55] Jesus is explaining that the forgiveness that we have received from God must bear fruit. Now, Galatians 5:22 and 23 lists the fruit of the Spirit, and forgiveness is not listed. Well, it is there in principle. You cannot forgive unless you have the Agape **love** in you. The fruit that are listed along with love include **peace**, **joy**,

---

51   New York Times (2008)
52   Luke 23:34 (King James Version)
53   King James Version
54   II Corinthians 3:17 (King James Version)
55   Matthew 6:14,15 (King James Version)

longsuffering, gentleness, goodness, faith, meekness, and **temperance,** which all emanate from *Agape love.*

When you forgive, however, it is not you who performs the forgiveness. It is the "God in you" that forgives. When you are willing to let the God in you forgive a person, God removes the unresolved hurts and pains out of your soul. Now that you are free, you can relate better in your relationships. You can use the virtue that you have received to restore other broken individuals. I have seen real life stories of parents who are in the courthouse waiting for their child's murderer to be sentenced, and have found that place of forgiveness. You would think they would lose their composure and try to attack the one who took their child from them. Instead, they pray for the murderer and try to forgive him. That's real forgiveness!

Now that you know what real forgiveness is, are there some people who you realize you have not forgiven? Describe what you thought forgiveness was and list the people you still need to forgive.

_____

_____

_____

_____

_____

_____

_____

_____

_____

_____

_____

_____

_____

_____

_____

_____

_____

_____

_____

_____

_____

_____

THIS WOMAN'S WORK

It's hard on a man. Now begins the craft of the Father.
(Kate Bush)

NOW THAT WE have discussed the dynamics of forgiveness, it is time to discuss the actual work of forgiveness. There are principles of forgiveness, and I will explain each one in depth. The seven steps of forgiveness are captured in the following acronym:

Faith

Offering

Remembering

Grieving

Irrigation

Ventilation

Expression

Step I: Faith

The first step in the forgiveness process is *faith*. This faith entails both a faith in GOD along with faith in the specific person(s) that GOD has anointed to help you through your process. Forgiveness is a spiritual gift, which means the gift comes from GOD. When you experience GOD's forgiveness, he gives you the responsibility to forgive others. Notice this word "responsibility." It is a combination of two words *response* and *ability*. Your response to GOD forgiving you is that you now have the ability and must use it to forgive others. Specifically, at the moment of salvation, the Holy Spirit dwells in the believer. Philippians 2:11 states, *"For it is GOD which dwelleth in us both to will and to do of His good pleasure."*[56] Hence, you can demonstrate your faith by allowing the Holy Spirit to work in and through you to forgive others. It is actually the Spirit that enables you to forgive, but the forgiveness won't happen unless you give Him permission. When you give the Holy Spirit permission to work in us to forgive, you are demonstrating faith in GOD. Now, if you truly have faith in GOD you also will demonstrate that faith towards the person that GOD has ordained to help you.

Many clients enter my office and assume that they randomly chose me. They saw my name as one of the providers in their insurance network and they randomly chose me. They soon realize that providence brought them into my office. Many clients come looking for medication as a temporary fix. However, what they find is spiritual guidance to help deliver them from their condition. This is important because if a client says that she has faith in GOD but will not trust the person GOD has sent to help her, then she will not receive the healing she so desperately needs. I tell my clients before we embark on this journey of forgiveness, "I am going to direct you to do things that may seem crazy, but unless you believe that this process is in your best interest, I will not be able to help you."

This first "faith" step is the most important of the seven steps because it is where the commitment begins. Right from the start, I ask for a commitment from every person who states that she is willing to go through this process. The reason is, when the process becomes

---

56   King James Version

painful, clients are tempted to quit, and many people do quit. I want them to count the cost of their commitment beforehand and still make a commitment to endure. When the temptation to quit comes, they can revert to their commitment rather than to their current feelings. This process is similar to having a healthy marriage. The commitment to endure the marriage for "richer and for poorer, through sickness and through health, unto death us do part" actually should occur before the marriage. If you have a pre-nuptial agreement or a divorce clause in your mind before you get married, you are laying the foundation for failure. Just like in marriage where one partner is really not committed to the marriage, some of my clients are not committed to the forgiveness process. However, just as GOD gives us a measure of faith to believe in Jesus for salvation, GOD can give you a measure of faith to believe in the healing process. Many Christians quote Isaiah, *"By His stripes we are healed,"*[57] but it takes faith to possess that which already belongs to you.

Step II: Offering

Now that faith in God and in the forgiveness process has been established, the next step involves rendering an *offering*, specifically a peace offering. In the Old Testament, a peace offering was given if the one giving the offering had met the prerequisite, which was to be in right standing with GOD. The peace offering was not to atone for one's sin, for atonement had already occurred. In the peace offering, the priest would sacrifice an unblemished animal (lamb or sheep) and the priest would sprinkle blood on the altar. The unblemished animal was a valuable thing to give up, and the animal had to die. One of the greatest things that humans value is their will. GOD gave us free will, and with this free will you can choose to put our faith in GOD or you can choose like Frank Sinatra said to do it "my way." For forgiveness to take place, this process must be led and controlled by the Holy Spirit.

---

57   Isaiah 53:5 (King James Version)

Your will has to die. This is precisely what is offered, your will. While this may sound somewhat simple, you will soon find out that letting go of your will is anything but simple. Encapsulated in your will are the resilience, the determination, the fight, the resolve, and your entire survival mechanism. Your will has functioned as your confidant, your best friend, and the one who has not let you down. When you were lied to, cheated on, abused, and disrespected, your will was always there to have your back and to strengthen you to go on. Now after all these years with your will, this best friend and confidant has to die. More specifically, you have to kill it. You must offer your will to GOD to be sacrificed. The reason why your will has to die is because it actually distracts and prevents you from reaching your destiny.

You see, forgiveness is not natural. Your will attempts to satisfy the flesh or your human nature. Forgiveness is not in your will's repertoire. It does not make logical sense to forgive someone who has hurt and abused you. Revenge makes logical sense. Your will constantly will lead you down a path that is in the best interest of your flesh rather than your spirit. That is why we must be led by the Holy Spirit. The Holy Spirit will not necessarily lead you down a path that is comfortable or painless, but He will lead you to the place where your life can give God the most glory and where you can find healing.

When Moses led the people of Israel out of Egypt, GOD specifically told Moses to go a circuitous route, which was the *long* way. One of GOD's reasons was that He knew the heart of the children of Israel. If they went in the direction of the Philistine camp, they would have frightened and would have returned to their bondage in Egypt. GOD knows the ending from the beginning and also knows how to take you where He has already predestined you to go. Even Jesus himself had to wrestle with His will. In the garden of Gethsemane, in so many words He said that if I could have it my way, I wouldn't be crucified. However, He offered His will to GOD and thus said, "*Nevertheless, not my will, but thine, be done.*"[58]

In the context of forgiveness, you have to do the same thing if you

---

58   Luke 22:42, King James Version

really want to experience true forgiveness. I tell my clients all the time, "If GOD ain't driving, HE ain't riding." Often times we want to be the driver and let GOD ride shotgun in the passenger seat. However, GOD does not want to ride with someone who does not know where he or she is going. To forgive you must surrender your will and let GOD's plan of forgiveness navigate your healing process.

Now that you know *what* to offer, it is time to discuss *how* you offer your will. This process is not a long, drawn out process; but consists of a simple and sincere prayer. You simply pray that GOD will accept your will as the thing to be sacrificed. Sincerely surrender your will to GOD. Even after you sacrifice your will, you will see vestiges of the old you trying to do things your way. This is part of the test. Be aware of this process, but continue to commit your ways unto the Lord. This notion of surrendering one's will to GOD is so vital to the forgiveness process. Cognitively, it makes sense, but when the time comes to actually let go and let GOD, many women just will not let go. I have facilitated numerous seminars on relationships, healing, and forgiveness, where I discuss the steps and the wisdom behind forgiveness, and everyone in the audience starts off excited. Then when it is time to act on what has been learned, the excitement immediately evaporates. When I ask, "Alright, who is ready to forgive their spouse?" you would have thought that I said someone died. They know they need to forgive, but they were not ready to forgive. For you to progress to the next stage, however, you have to be ready and willing to forgive and do so.

Step III: Remembering

I know you have heard the phrase, "forgive and forget." The reality is that during the process of forgiveness, and even when forgiveness is accomplished, we still can, and do, remember the hurts and pain. GOD has given us a wonderful brain that rarely forgets anything. As mentioned earlier, even when we are subjected to intense trauma and have amnesia, the brain is still able to retrieve almost all memories. This process is analogous to deleting files from a computer. Even after you push the delete button and permanently delete files, any good IT person is able to find them. So, we really do not forget the hurt, the abandonment, the abuse, the lies, or the rejection. The difference is that after we have completed the process of forgiveness, remembering is not painful. During the process of forgiveness, however, remembering is extremely painful because the one who is remembering is now confronting the raw feelings that she has avoided for so long. A common fear with this step of remembering is the uncertainty of opening "Pandora's Box." The fear is that when I allow myself to experience the suppressed feelings, I may have a breakdown. The truth of the matter is that is a realistic fear. There is a potential that the suppressed feelings can overtake the person. That is why this process should be facilitated by an experienced and trained practitioner.

During the initial interview process, I ask my clients to identify the seven people that have hurt them the most. Sometimes the list is shorter, and sometimes the list is longer. Often times, many of my clients forget or do not know that they themselves must be on the list. Who the client will remember first depends who is on the list. More often than not, the client is last on the list. This process of remembering is very important in the forgiveness process. Remembering takes the suppressed feelings and brings them to the forefront so they can be expressed. Remembering involves going back and uprooting the emotional details of major hurts and pains. It involves you recalling the sometimes ugly names that influential people in your life called you. You may have been called fat, stupid, ho, bi—h, ugly, slut, mean, or a mistake. You need to remember how it felt to hear that. You need to remember the abuse, the molestation, the rape, the violence, and the neglect. Now, it is common for people to avoid the pain in remembering by making the process cognitive rather than emotional. Hence, they look at these events from a historical perspective trying to put the pieces of the puzzle together rather than emoting and expressing the tremendous hurt. However, it is vitally important to emote while remembering. I encourage clients to say "I felt" instead of "I think."

Another tactic to minimize the pain is to rationalize or make excuses for why things happened the way they did. I often hear, "my mother got treated the same way from her mother, so I understand." While some of the statements and assessments are true, they facilitate deviation from the process of expressing suppressed hurts and pains. I insist that clients do not defend or make excuses during the remembering phase for the persons that hurt them. They need to express the emotions just as they first felt them. At the moment your mother called you a derogatory name, you did not immediately think to yourself, "She got this behavior from her mother." No, you immediately felt hurt and rejection. This raw pain needs to be expressed just as it was initially felt. As mentioned earlier, hurts and pain can progress into anger, rage, wrath, and malice. Even during the remembering phase, if you express anger, you still must express the raw hurt for the pain to be expressed successfully. Because these unresolved and unexpressed feelings have remained inside of you for years, it is not easy to part with them.

Step IV: Grieving

The process of forgiveness involves releasing emotions, dependencies, and strongholds. Most people think that because the emotions and the traumatic experiences are so painful, it would be easy to release them. On the contrary, the difficulty in letting these feelings go is analogous to a battered wife leaving her abusive husband. Despite the constant abuse, attacks, and agonizing pain that a battered woman experiences, she and many others like her would rather stay with the "devil she knows" than to venture out to find a peace that seems unknown. Therefore, considerable attention and energy must be devoted to the grieving process. The painful experiences and the emotional dependence on them need to die. Actually, they need to be killed. The earlier process of *remembering* was supposed to kill these emotions and dependence on them. This fourth stage accomplishes the process of grieving and bringing closure to the past. When a loved one or someone you have depended on for so long dies, the grieving process can be very difficult. You ask yourself, "How am I going to make it without him or her?" If you grieve properly, you can go on with your life not depending on the person or the memory to get you through. There is no definitive timetable for grieving, but most if not all people go through similar stages of grieving.

Kubler-Ross[59] described the process of grieving with death and dying in five steps:

1. Denial
2. Anger
3. Bargaining
4. Depression
5. Acceptance

Many women get stuck in the anger phase of the grieving process. There is resentment and anger for letting go of the emotions which were so much a part of them. This is usually when some clients stop coming to counseling. This is the most difficult of all the steps, yet it accounts for the greatest progress in the forgiveness process when complete. It is no accident that grieving is the fourth step out of seven. Steps one through three are analogous to traveling on level ground. When you get to step four, it functions like a hill or an incline. You need to exert energy to climb to the top of the hill. Once you get to the top, however, it is downhill the rest of the way. I have often asked people what was their greatest fear. Many say that their greatest fear is having a loved one on whom they depend dies. Without prompting, they immediately say, "I don't know if I could make it without him/ her." That's how many women feel about the loss of their will or the loss of control. They say, "I can't imagine my life without the security of being in control."

---

59   Elizabeth Kubler-Ross ("On Death & Dying 1969)

Those clinicians who are gifted in grief work understand that the client needs to get to the place where he or she accepts the death. You do not need to avoid thinking about the person who died, rather grow to be at peace with the reality of their death. Instead of thinking that you can't make it with out them or asking them, "Why did you leave me?" focus on the good that they brought while they were alive. Furthermore, the clinician helps the client to understand how to take that good and invest it in his/her future. So instead of looking back, the client has accepted the death and now is looking forward. Specifically, as it relates to grieving one's will, you should celebrate the great things that your will did for you. I remind clients that it was actually healthy for you to take matters into your own hands when people had continually let you down. If everyone you trust takes advantage of you, uses you, abuses you, or neglects you, it is wise to take your trust and dependence from them and focus on yourself. Some theologians may criticize this technique because they may believe you should put your focus on GOD instead of yourself. The two concepts, however, are not mutually exclusive. Well, the truth of the matter is that GOD intended for humans to reflect the love of GOD in a natural way. The mother is supposed to be the first reflection of love for a newborn baby. When parents and supposed loved ones reflect evil instead of good, the true light of GOD is very difficult to see. GOD often appears evil and uncaring. Hence, the first step in this circumstance is to take the free will that GOD gave you and seek shelter, even if that shelter is you! Then, when your will takes you as far as it can go, sacrifice it and learn how to depend on GOD instead.

Step V: Irrigation

Stacy seemed to have cruised through her forgiveness process. She was diligent in remembering and diligent in grieving. I asked her how she felt about her ex-boyfriend. She declared, "I am at peace with him. I am no longer enslaved by what he did to me." I asked her about her parents, and she replied in a similar fashion. I even asked

Stacy to describe how she felt about the mistakes she has made. She replied, "It was definitely hard to forgive myself and to let go of the guilt, but I did, and I feel good." I then asked her about the last person she was supposed to forgive. When I asked, "How do you feel about the woman who slept with your husband? What is her name?" Stacy's face went blank, and so did her mind. She tried to remember the woman's name but she could not. I immediately knew that she had buried that hurt way beneath the surface. She had yet to really tap into the raw emotion that she had denied. Stacy thought she was over that trauma. I told Stacy to return to the *remembering* phase until she remembered the woman's name was. Although our next session was not until the following week, a hysterical Stacy called me the next day asking to meet that day. When she came into my office, she stated, "She deserves to die for what she did." Stacy really was not homicidal, but she allowed herself to express the tremendous hurt that had progressed into wrath.

Irrigation in the context of forgiveness involves the process by which the soul is intentionally flooded with memories relating to the remembering phase to determine if there are any vestiges of unforgiveness. Deeply suppressed pain creates the illusion that forgiveness has already taken place. Just as irrigation is used to clean a wound by applying water or a medicated solution, irrigation in the context of forgiveness involves applying focused insight to clean any remnants of unforgiveness.

Step VI: Ventilation:

Ventilation is the process of supplying fresh air and eliminating foul air. As it relates to forgiveness, ventilation occurs when the lid of the soul is opened. Imagine a soda bottle being shaken vigorously. The soda moves towards the top of the bottle desiring to escape. If there is a cap on the bottle, then there is no place for the soda to go but to settle back down in the bottle. Likewise, the same process exists for emotions. The traumas and stressors of life often shake you up like soda in a bottle. You feel pain which progresses to anger, and sometimes to rage or wrath. That is when you feel we need to "vent" or get some things off your chest. Specifically, ventilation is the process where you confront those who have hurt you so that forgiveness can occur.

Forgiveness is a legal decision. For there to be a pardon, an acquittal, or a ruling of forgiveness, charges first must be brought. These charges are presented as specific violations of the law. If you are ignorant of the law, you may not know that you are being violated. Many women have their boundaries violated all the time. The unfortunate tragedy is that often they don't realize that they are being violated. Every client of mine going through the process of forgiveness must confront with specificity the perpetrators and their specific offenses. You must confront the perpetrators of the offenses without making any excuses for them. If the perpetrators are deceased or their address is unknown, then it is recommended that you write a letter to confront them. This confrontation is not just legal or factual, but it is primarily emotional. I usually invite the parent, spouse, or whomever needs to be forgiven to the session to for the confrontation. Invariably, when the confrontation is over, the response from my clients is "I feel lighter and relieved," as if their deep-seated burdens just melted away.

Step VII: Expression

The seventh and final step in the forgiveness process is expression. The one needing to forgive has to do two final things: believe and receive. Remember, forgiveness is a gift from GOD, and it is a spiritual gift. Because it is spiritual, you can only receive it by faith. Specifically, in this stage you have to pray that God will work the effectual work forgiveness, and by faith, expect that God will accomplish it. When you sense that the power of GOD has made a definitive change in you regarding forgiveness, you need to express that it aloud. You should communicate to the people you are forgiving that they are forgiven. Specifically, the expression of forgiveness involves a declaration. The one who is forgiving should declare, "I forgive you." Sometimes this step can be accomplished in person, and sometimes over the phone. Sometimes it can be done by speaking to yourself. You must declare it aloud so you can hear it. Finally, there should be an expression of thanksgiving to GOD who wrought this work of forgiveness in and through you.

Are you willing to complete this process? Describe what you learned about forgiveness that you didn't know before.

_____

_____

_____

_____

_____

_____

_____

_____

_____

_____

_____

_____

_____

_____

_____

_____

_____

_____

_____

The Proof is in the Peace

Free at last, free at last; thank GOD Almighty I am free at last. (Dr. Martin Luther King)

Therefore, having been justified by faith, we have peace with God through our Lord Jesus Christ.[60]

KIMBERLY CANNOT BELIEVE how good she feels. After completing the journey of forgiveness, she now is free. Free from the weight, free from the guilt, and free from the pain. She does not have amnesia. She has not forgotten the people that hurt her, but when she happens to be reminded of them, there is peace that seems to surpass understanding and a joy that is unspeakable. She finds herself often smiling probably appearing crazy in public. She feels lighter, and she has lost a tremendous amount of emotional weight without trying Weight Watchers or Jenny Craig. People wonder why she is smiling and to whom is she speaking? She is talking to God and to the *new* Kimberly. She is smiling because life now has meaning and it is wonderful. She is grateful for what God has wrought in her life. As she walks past her favorite fast food restaurant, she does not feel compelled to stop and gratify an emotional urge. She now realizes that she does not need to cope by using earthly things since she has experienced and expressed an eternal process called forgiveness.

---

60   Romans 5:1 (King James Version)

Now it is important to understand that peace, and peace alone, is the evidence that real forgiveness has taken place. Many people erroneously use the status of a relationship as a barometer to know whether they have forgiven the ones who have offended them. Peace is the proof of forgiveness, but peace is not the absence of conflict.

Many people come into my office and swear that they have forgiven people based on how they get along better than before. I commend them on the progress but explain to them that the absence of conflict does not constitute proof of forgiveness. Forgiveness does not mean you have a great relationship with the one you believe you have just forgiven. As a matter of fact, it is usually the opposite. Many people pretend to have a great relationship while deceiving themselves and others. I repeatedly tell my clients that just because I forgive people does not mean I trust them. Forgiveness simply emancipates me from the burden and grip that their offense had on me. When I forgive, I have peace within myself and with them. However, I am not foolish to assume that everything is perfect between us; rather, it probably behooves me to create some distance and to establish some boundaries. Again, the proof is in the peace you experience. If you reflect on a relationship and you still have traces of anger, resentment, bitterness, or regret towards the offender, than you have not forgiven the offender. If you are still making excuses for the perpetrator, then you have not forgiven him.

Forgiveness not only gives you peace so that you feel better, but it empowers you to do better. Where there is unforgiveness, there are the patterns of behavior learned from the perpetrators. For example, though the children of Israel had been delivered from Egyptian bondage, many still had a bondage mentality. When they encountered conflict or disappointment, they longed to back to their slavery experience. Similarly, many women have had terrible upbringings, and as soon as they are old enough, they leave home. While they leave the home, they often do not leave the dysfunction which occurred in the home. For example, many mothers who stayed in abusive relationships with their husbands or boyfriends either consciously or unconsciously taught their sons and daughters to be protectors by: 1) subjecting them to vulnerable conditions, and 2) encouraging them to lie or to get help from the police or others. This creates a personality pattern in a child to always be in a posture of fixing people who are vulnerable. This leads women to be attracted to abusive, emotionally needy, and dysfunctional men. That unhealthy pattern of thinking and relating was taught and learned while in the home. Even if you completely detest the environment, if you do not unlearn what you were taught and learn something new, you will replicate those patterns of thinking, feeling, and behaving. With the process of forgiveness comes the recognition that those patterns were hurtful, unhealthy, and sinful. When one forgives, there is a conscious decision to learn new values and new patterns of living. After forgiveness has taken place, you experience greater insight into the depth of the generational patterns which in turn further the experience of peace.

Every Christian was born an enemy to God. We came into the world already violating His law. This resulted in God having wrath. The Bible says that *"the wages of sin is death."*[61] Furthermore, the bible also says that God's wrath comes on the children of disobedience.[62] Jesus, however, satisfied the wrath of God when He lived a perfect life, shed His blood, died, was buried, and was resurrected for our justification. Jesus paid the penalty for our sins and purchased our forgiveness. Hence, when one receives God's grace and mercy and places her faith in Jesus alone for salvation, she is completely forgiven. The result of this transaction is called justification. You are declared right with God or in right standing with God. This declaration brings peace. The peace is the evidence that true forgiveness has occurred.

When you marvel at how you are no longer angry, anxious, or overwhelmed, and you are able to reflect on your painful past in great detail and yet have peace, you have successfully completed the forgiveness diet. Enjoy the *new you!* Now, this diet isn't just for weight loss, but also to keep the weight off. This diet must be a daily

61   Romans 6:23a(King James Version)
62   Colossians 3:6 (King James Version)

diet where you address hurts and pains immediately and not suppress them. This new lifestyle is both preventative and also for maintenance. It contributes to the prevention of emotional and physical diseases, while simultaneously maintaining your current health. Remember, not only have grudges been dissolved during this process, but also patterns of unhealthy thinking have been corrected. During periods of weakness, you may be tempted to regress and return to old ways of thinking, feeling, and behaving. I want to encourage you to *keep your eyes on the prize* and *press toward the mark for the prize of the high calling in Christ Jesus.*[63]

---

63   Philippians 3:14 (King James Version)

Describe how you feel. Are you ready to really begin this forgiveness diet? Describe why.

_____

_____

_____

_____

_____

_____

_____

_____

_____

_____

_____

_____

_____

_____

_____

_____

_____

_____

_____

_____

_____

_____

_____

CPSIA information can be obtained at www.ICGtesting.com
Printed in the USA
LVOW101250101111

254361LV00002B/23/P